CANCER:

My Enemy, My Friend

Preface

'If no untimely fate awaits it, Singapore promises to become the
emporium and pride of the East.'

Sir Stamford Raffles, 1823

For many travellers, arriving nowadays by air, Singapore provides
their first exciting glimpse of the East. In earlier times, a visitor
coming from Europe or America by ship would already have called at
one or more Eastern ports along the way. Yet arrival at Singapore
always made a vivid impression.

An Englishman, gazing from the deck as his steamer approached the
wharf, noted: "There Malay jostles Chinaman, Kling rubs shoulders
with Javanese, Arab elbows Seedy-boy, and Dyak stares at Bugis, all
their dirty bodies swathed either in nothing to speak of, or else in
scarlet and yellow and blue and gold . . ." That was in the 1890s.

A century later, Singapore continues to make an indelible impression on new arrivals who unexpectedly find they have come to a city
more modern than the ones they have left behind. Despite the
"untimely fate" which indeed befell the city in 1942, Singapore has
survived and prospered to fulfil the most optimistic dreams of its
founder. Where godowns and shophouses once lined the waterfront,
commercial palaces of concrete and glass now reach up to the sky.

But, for visitors (and residents) who understand the value of roots,
and so care about things past, there *are* sights to be seen which have
not altered much in a hundred years: certain streets, buildings and
even some passers-by seem imbued still with the authentic spirit of
Conrad and Maugham.

It is for readers of this sort that *Travellers' Tales* has now been
enlarged and republished. Here they will find the personal, human
experiences which others, much like themselves, enjoyed or suffered

in the Singapore of former days: as they pushed through motley crowds along the five-foot ways; tried to make themselves understood while exploring markets, temples and mosques; attended wedding celebrations and strange festivals; mastered their first practical lessons in the oriental art of bargaining; found themselves, by intent or otherwise, in red-light districts; coped on a daily basis with heat, insects, unfamiliar food and unfamiliar bathrooms – and took Dutch Wives into their beds! This is time travel at its very best.

M.W. 1996

Contents

7

Tale-end

Illustrations

LKC	Lim Kheng Chye
ATKG	Andrew Tan Kim Guan
PYKM	Paul Yap Kong Meng
Archives	Archives & Oral History Department, Singapore

In Anno 1703, I called at *Johore* in my Way to *China*, and he [the Sultan] treated me very kindly, and made me a Present of the Island of *Sincapure*, but I told him it could be of no Use to a private Person, tho' a proper Place for a Company to settle a Colony on, lying in the Centre of Trade, and being accommodated with good Rivers and safe Harbours, so conveniently situated, that all Winds served Shipping both to go out and come into those Rivers.

ALEXANDER HAMILTON
A New Account of the East Indies (1727)

1819

Skulls on the Sand

*When Singapore was founded by Sir Stamford Raffles in 1819
Abdullah bin Abdul Kadir was only twenty-two. He came to Singapore to make a living as interpreter, language teacher and, on occasion,
as private secretary to Raffles. These extracts from Abdullah's autobiography describe the very early days when Colonel William Farquhar
was helping Raffles to develop the new settlement of Singapore.*

Now at this time the seas round Singapore, so far from being navigated freely by men, were feared even by jinns and devils, for along
the shores were the sleeping-huts of the pirates. Whenever they plundered
a ship or a ketch or a cargo-boat, they brought it in to Singapore
where they shared the spoils and slaughtered the crew, or fought to
the death among themselves to secure their gains.

The Sea Gypsies in their boats behaved like wild animals. Whenever
they saw a crowd of people coming, if there was time they made off
quickly in their boats: if there was not time they leapt into the sea
and swam under water like fish, disappearing from view for about half
an hour before coming to the surface as much as a thousand yards
away from the place where they entered the water. Both the men and
women behaved like this. As for their children words fail me. Whenever they saw anybody they would scream as though death was upon
them, like someone who catches sight of a tiger. All these people
brought fish for the Temenggong to eat. None of them knew any
way of catching fish except by spearing them. The fish most frequently
caught by spear was the *tenggiri* though occasionally they would get
other kinds, for instance dorabs. . . .

The Temenggong ordered the Sea Gypsies to sell fish to Colonel
Farquhar's men. Although they did come bearing fish it was with great
reluctance, and they were astonished at the sight of the tents and
men wearing clothes and so on. Whatever price was offered for the

13

fish, or if it was bartered for a little tobacco or rice, they would take it and go away. Whenever they came Colonel Farquhar gave them money and clothes and rice to make them more amenable, for he saw that they wore no clothes. After this had gone on for a day or two they became fearless enough to rub shoulders with the newcomers. Only the children remained wild, to such an extent they became ill with fright at the sight of people. One child was even drowned at sea off Telok Ayer because he was so frightened when several men walked near his boat that he instantly jumped into the water, at the time when it was high tide. They waited but he did not appear again, and was lost after being carried out to sea by the current. . . .

All along the shore there were hundreds of human skulls rolling about on the sand; some old, some new, some with hair still sticking to them, some with the teeth filed and others without. News of these skulls was brought to Colonel Farquhar and when he had seen them he ordered them to be gathered up and cast into the sea. So the people collected them in sacks and threw them into the sea. The Sea Gypsies were asked "Whose are all these skulls?" and they replied "These are the skulls of men who were robbed at sea. They were slaughtered here. Wherever a fleet of boats or a ship is plundered it is brought to this place for a division of the spoils. Sometimes there is wholesale slaughter among the crews when the cargo is grabbed. Sometimes the pirates tie people up and try out their weapons here along the sea shore." Here too was the place where they went in for cock-fighting and gambling.

One day Colonel Farquhar wanted to ascend the Forbidden Hill, as it was called by the Temenggong. The Temenggong's men said "None of us have the courage to go up the hill because there are many ghosts on it. Every day one can hear on it sounds as of hundreds of men. Sometimes one hears the sound of heavy drums and of people shouting." Colonel Farquhar laughed and said, "I should like to see your ghosts" and turning to his Malacca men "Draw this gun to the top of the hill." Among them there were several who were frightened, but having no option they pulled the gun up. All who went up were Malacca men, none of the Singapore men daring to approach the hill. On the hill there was not much forest and not many large trees, only a few shrubs here and there. Although the men were frightened they were shamed by the presence of Colonel Farquhar and went up whether they wanted to or not. When they reached the top Colonel Farquhar ordered the gun to be loaded and then he himself fired twelve rounds in succession over the top of the hill in front of them. Then he ordered a pole to be erected on which he hoisted the English flag. He said "Cut down all these bushes." He also ordered them to make a path for people to go up and down the hill. Everyday there was this work being done, the undergrowth being slashed down and a pathway cleared.

At that time there were few animals, wild or tame on the Island of Singapore, except rats. There were thousands of rats all over the district, some almost as large as cats. They were so big that they used to attack us if we went out walking at night and many people were knocked over. In the house where I was living we used to keep a cat. One night at about midnight we heard the cat mewing, and my friend went out carrying a light to see why the cat was making such a noise. He saw six or seven rats crowding round and biting the cat; some bit its ears, some its paws, some its nose so that it could no longer move but only utter cry after cry. When my companion saw what was happening he shouted to me and I ran out at the back to have a look. Six or seven men came pressing round to watch but did nothing to release the cat, which only cried the louder at the sight of so many men, like a person beseeching help. Then someone fetched a stick and struck at the rats, killing the two which were biting the cat's ears. Its ears freed, the cat then pounced on another rat and killed it. Another was hit by the man with a stick and the rest ran away. The cat's face and nose were lacerated and covered with blood. This was the state of affairs in all the houses, which were full of rats. They could hardly be kept under control, and the time had come when they took notice of people. Colonel Farquhar's place was also in the same state and he made an order saying "To anyone who kills a rat I will give one *wang*." When people heard of this they devised all manner of instruments for killing rats. Some made spring-traps, some pincer-traps, some cage-traps, some traps with running nooses, some traps with closing doors, others laid poison or put down lime. I had never in my life before seen rats caught by liming; only now for the first time. Some searched for rat-holes, some speared the rats or killed them in various other ways. Every day crowds of people brought the dead bodies to Colonel Farquhar's place, some having fifty or sixty others only six or seven. At first the rats brought in every morning were counted almost in thousands, and Colonel Farquhar paid out according to his promise. After six or seven days a multitude of rats were still to be seen, and he promised five *duit* for each rat caught.

They were still brought in in thousands and Colonel Farquhar ordered a very deep trench to be dug and the dead bodies to be buried. So the numbers began to dwindle, until people were bringing in only some ten or twenty a day. Finally the uproar and the campaign against the rats in Singapore came to an end, the infestation having completely subsided.

Some time later a great many centipedes appeared, people being bitten by them all over the place. In every dwelling, if one sat for any length of time, two or three centipedes would drop from the attap roof. Rising in the morning from a night's sleep one would be sure to find two or three very large centipedes under one's mat, and they caused people much annoyance. When the news reached Colonel Farquhar he made an order saying that to anyone who killed a centipede he would give one *wang*. Hearing this people searched high and low for centipedes, and every day they brought in hundreds which they had caught by methods of their own devising. So the numbers dwindled until once in two or three days some twenty or thirty centipedes were brought in. Finally the campaign and furore caused by the centipedes came to an end, and people no longer cried out because of the pain when they got bitten. . . .

There is a story about how Mr. Raffles and Colonel Farquhar together debated the best way to enlarge the Settlement. Colonel Farquhar considered that Kampong Gelam should become the business quarter, that is to say a tradings centre with markets and so forth. But Mr. Raffles thought that the business quarter should be on the near side of the river. Colonel Farquhar said "This side is very unsuitable as the ground is all muddy and the water is not good. It will be very costly to reclaim the land. Besides, where can we obtain sufficient earth for banking?" Mr. Raffles replied "If Kampong Gelam were to become a business area this side of the river would remain unimproved for as long as a hundred years." Each of the two men held firmly to his own opinion, the one saying this the other that, each trying to find support for his view. They thought the matter over for three days. Then it occurred to Mr. Raffles that the small hill near Tanjong Singapura might be broken up and the earth used for banking on the near side of the river. The next day the two of them considered this idea and agreed to it. . . .

After three or four months the hill was flattened out and all the muddy pools, narrow water-channels and swampy ground were levelled off. There remained a few huge rocks, some as tall as elephants, and others even larger. These rocks were very useful, for the Chinese came in scores and broke them up for house building. There was no payment for the work, for everyone rushed to ask for the stone which was just given away.

It was then that they found at the point of the headland a rock lying in the bushes. The rock was smooth, about six feet wide, square in shape, and its face was covered with a chiselled inscription. But although it had writing this was illegible because of extensive scouring by water. Allah alone knows how many thousands of years old it may have been. After its discovery crowds of all races came to see it. The Indians declared that the writing was Hindu but they were unable to read it. The Chinese claimed that it was in Chinese characters. I went with a party of people, and also Mr. Raffles and Mr. Thomsen, and we all looked at the rock. I noticed that in shape the lettering was rather like Arabic, but I could not read it because owing to its great age the relief was partly effaced.

Many learned men came and tried to read it. Some brought flour-paste which they pressed on the inscription and took a cast, others rubbed lamp-black on it to make the lettering visible. But for all that they exhausted their ingenuity in trying to find out what language the letters represented they reached no decision. There the stone rested until recently with its inscription in relief. It was Mr. Raffles's opinion that the writing must be Hindu because the Hindus were the oldest of all immigrant races in the East, reaching Java and Bali and Siam, the inhabitants of which are all descended from them. However, not a single person in all Singapore was able to interpret the words chiselled on the rock. Allah alone knows. . . .

At the time when they were auctioning land Mr. Raffles said to me "You should take up four or five pieces of land here, for in the future the place may become densely populated." I replied "Sir, where can I get money enough to pay the price of the land, for I notice that a single piece of land sells for as much as $1,200 or $1,150 and how shall I find the money to build a stone house?" Mr. Raffles smiled when he heard my words and said "Don't you worry about money. You can settle that later, as long as you take the land first." But in my stupidity and ignorance I thought that if perchance I should run into debt it might be difficult for me to return when I wished to Malacca. And at that time it was easy enough to make money in Singapore. It was my practice to return home to Malacca for six months at a time and I thought that if I acquired land and built a

17

house I should certainly not be able to go back there. Moreover, I did not believe for a moment that Singapore could become so densely populated, nor did I realize that the land was being auctioned for nothing, no money being taken. It was an auction in name only. Later I saw that in selling in this way Mr. Raffles was being very shrewd, for if the land were merely given away free it would be grabbed by poor men who might never be able to afford to build houses of stone. Therefore the lots were auctioned for a high price so that only rich men would buy and they would build quickly. So it came about that because of my lack of foresight and my stupidity I did not follow Mr. Raffles's advice when he told me to take up land, and now I regret my mistake. But to what purpose, for as the Malays say "Realize your mistake in time and you may still gain something, realize it too late and you gain nothing.". . .

After that Mr. Raffles moved house to the top of Bukit Larangan (The Forbidden Hill) because many white men came wanting to put up houses. Instructions were given to clear the ground all round the hill. The men came across many fruit-trees as large as durian trees, six feet or more round the trunk. But owing to their great age their fruits were no larger than a durian just after the flower has faded. There were *dukus*, and lime trees and pomelo trees with fruit no larger than dwarf lime, and many other kinds of fruit like *langsat*, and fruits with a bad smell like those of the *pětai* and *jěring*. . . .

One morning Colonel Farquhar went for a walk by the side of Rochore River taking his dog with him. The dog took to the water in the river when suddenly it was seized by a crocodile. A moment later Colonel Farquhar was told that his dog had been eaten by a crocodile, and he ordered the men who were there to put up a dam blocking the river. The crocodile was hemmed in by the obstruction and speared to death. It was fifteen feet long. This was the first time that people realized there were crocodiles in Singapore. Colonel Farquhar ordered the crocodile's carcass to be brought along, and he hung it on a fig tree by the side of the Beras Basah river.

ABDULLAH BIN ABDUL KADIR
The Hikayat Abdullah (1849)
Trans. A.H. Hill

1824

The Fate of Singapore

As a Dutch officer, Colonel Nahuijs felt a sense of national grievance about the British settlement on Singapore. Communications were slow, and it seems clear from this letter (dated 10 June 1824) that word had not yet reached him about the Treaty, signed in London three months previously, in which the Dutch had formally withdrawn their objections to British occupation.

I believe that no person with any feeling can help being impressed when setting foot in Singapore, because he can now see as a seat of European trade and industry a place which only five years before was a cavern and hiding place for murderers and pirates. This impression, it is true, is considerably dimmed for the Hollander by the thought that the English are settled in a place to which only his nation had a right, but as a friend of humanity, he must prefer seeing this island in the possession of civilized Christians to it being in the hands of pirates and murderers who made the journey through the Straits of Malacca exceedingly dangerous. And, let me ask you, would Singapore not still have been to this date the same den of murderers as it was in the past had it not been taken over by the English? . . .

As a Hollander I regret that we ourselves did not wrest Singapore out of the hands of these pirates instead of leaving them in the possession of this island which we are now disputing with the English nation. But enough of this.

The island of Singapore, separated from the mainland of Johore by a very narrow strait, is nearly thirty English miles long from east to west and twenty-one broad from north to south. The climate is healthy, but very warm, the thermometer at mid-day mostly registering from 86° to 92°. The drinking water is very good, but, especially in

the case of lengthy droughts, of insufficient quantity to supply many
ships at the same time. For this reason reservoirs or rain-troughs
were being constructed. The soil seems to be suitable for the planting
of pepper and gambier, but not for coffee. Before the occupation
of Singapore by the English, some Chinese living a few miles inland
earned a livelihood by planting and preparing the gambier.

Ground standing vacant is obtainable by any person without payment whatsover. Anyone desiring it simply applied to the Resident,
who thereupon issued a grant free of charge, unless the ground was
owned or occupied by natives, in which case it was necessary to make
an agreement regarding the transfer with the natives beforehand.

The land is mostly hilly and is thickly covered with trees. Many of
the hills in the neighbourhood of the beach are already adorned with
houses of various Europeans... The house of the Resident also
stands on such a hill. From it one has the best view of the Roads,
the Straits of Singapore and the Straits of Malacca, as well as the
neighbouring islands. The house itself, however, did not attract me
very much and seemed very cramped...

The houses of the settlers or traders are close to the shore and are
well built. Most of them are raised high above the ground and roofed
with stone tiles, which are partly brought from Malacca and partly
from China.

Most of the houses are on the left bank of the river, which divides
the town into two parts. A few are on the right bank, where the
Chinese and Arab settlement containing more than one hundred
good houses is situated. There is a good bridge over the river 200
feet long and 32 feet broad.

Singapore can already boast of about thirty tastefully built European
houses. These are placed a short distance from one another and in
front of them runs a carriage-way, which they all make use of in the
afternoons. This riding and driving appears to me to be very similar
to riding around in a riding-school, because one has to go round
the same circular road four or five times in an afternoon in order to
make a tour worth the name. ....

Many servants and coolies are Chinese, whose number totals about
5,000; most of them are occupied in agriculture. The Malays seldom
work for the Europeans; they are too lazy and indolent by nature
to devote themselves to a definitely daily task. The Malays settled in
Singapore for the most part submit to the so-called Malayan Tommagung, the former head of the pirates, whom the British government

support with a monthly payment of Sp. Piaster 700. In addition to this income of Sp. Piaster 700 per month he also enjoys certain revenue arising out of the ferrying across the river and some small charges which he levies on native vehicles and on the cutting of timber. This Tommagung is generally said to have a very good understanding with his elder brothers the pirates and to maintain an active correspondence with them, giving them regular news of the comings and goings in Singapore harbour and the destination, cargo and strength of the different ships. The Tommagung lives with his dependents a short distance away from the European town on a site alotted to him by the British government of Singapore, on account of the frequent quarrels and murders for which his dependents have been responsible.

Over all these people as well as over the Bouginese settled in Singapore, the British Resident has not the least authority, even when they attack the Europeans . . .

Two companies of Bengalese and a detachment of 25 European Artillery must hardly suffice to ensure the safety of their people and the large values which are lying in Singapore warehouses in the way of goods, especially opium and piece work, two valuable articles which the natives particularly prize. Many of the residents are not without anxiety that a man like the Malayan Tommagung, tempted by the large treasure, could easily be induced with the underlings and a great many of his friends the pirates, to attack the weak garrison and citizens unexpectedly and then clear off with his booty to places where he could not easily be traced. People were hoping therefore that a good fort would be built, that the garrison would be strengthened and the port guarded by a couple of the Company's cruisers from Bombay.

As a measure of precaution the British government after the minor dispute with the natives have ordained that nobody other than of high rank, whose names must be registered at the police station shall have the right to go about within the European establishment carrying a kris or other weapon. . . .

In the fundamental laws which were laid down by Sir Stamford Raffles on the foundation of Singapore all gambling, without exception, was forbidden and it was assumed that this would never be permitted, even though farmed out. The leasing of the dice gambling by the Resident has put up the backs of most of the good settlers, especially the magistrates, of whom many have tendered their resignation. . . .

Another circumstance which makes the settlers in a sense dissatisfied with the present Resident is that he is very economical and saving with the country's funds and undertakes few public works in contrast with Lieutenant-Governor Raffles, who was not very sparing with Government money and laid it out for the public benefit and for the improvement of Singapore. So long as the fate of Singapore is undecided and it is still uncertain whether that establishment is to remain in the hands of the English it seems to me cautious and sensible not to lay out too much money on this insecure possession.

"Extracts from the letters of Col. Nahuijs"
Trans. H.E. Miller
*Journal of the Malayan Branch, Royal
Asiatic Society*, Vol. XIX. II. 1941

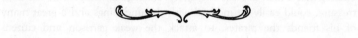

1824

The Flag on the Hill

In the old days, many young men came out to Singapore in search of adventure and fortune. Among them was Walter Scott Duncan who arrived in Singapore four years after its founding and got a job as a merchant's clerk with A.L. Johnston & Co. Duncan's diary is one of the earliest accounts of life in Singapore during the pioneer years.

April 15th. – Went off to the *Hastings* about half-past seven. Found that Dr. Montgomerie and Mr. Barnard were expected.... Waited till near 9, when dreading something had occurred to detain them, we were on the point of sitting down to breakfast, when a boat answering the description of the one I had seen made her appearance among the junks making towards us. On approaching a little nearer saw there were about 5 to 6 Europeans seated in the stern. Orders were instantly issued to the cook to prepare something additional to meet the consumption of as many additional mouths.... The heat very great, much so that one or two were obliged to leave the table in the poop, ere we had done eating....

April 16th. – ... This had been a gloomy and threatening day, and fatal I am sorry to add to three unfortunate Malays who were struck dead by lightning at Kampong Gelam about 2 p.m. A boy was likewise much hurt. The thunder was sharp and extremely close, the sky exceedingly clouded, but not followed by much rain. Alongside of the *Hastings* at 20 minutes past 4 p.m. Sate down to table 10 in number, including the Captain and Chief Mate. Had an excellent dinner prepared.... Landed about 9. Went in to Mr. Guthrie's and had a glass of brandy and water.

April 17th. – To-day arrived the American brig *Leander*, Capt. Roundy from Batavia. Having waited so long for a vessel from the place in the expectation of getting dispatches, our disappointment may be easily

23

guessed at on finding we were fated yet to wait some time longer. . . . Brings accounts of the ship in which Sir T. S. Raffles had embarked all his collection of natural curiosities, the finest ever made in this quarter of the world, all his valuable manuscripts, furniture, wardrobe, and whatever he intended taking home, – having sunk in Bencoolen roads, only a few hours previous to the time he had fixed for his own and Lady Raffles' embarkation, and so very suddenly that the people on board had barely time to save their lives; to save aught else was out of the question. . . .

April 20th. – In the morning a ship at anchor in the roads which we hoped to be the *Fazil Currim*, but which afterward turned out to be the *Good Hope* . . .

In the evening a brig in sight to the eastward, for whom the flag on the hill had been flying through the greater part of the day. Went down from Mr. Read's a little while before 8 p.m. to make enquiries after her, and on landing at the godown wharf found the Capt. of the brig had just arrived before me, that he was from Batavia and had brought a good many letters. Busy assorting immediately. Only one for myself, from T. Bain. Collected those directed for Mr. and Mrs. Read, and set off to his house to deliver them to him, mostly Europe letters. He received them with singular coolness and composure. Sate down until I had finished reading Rt. Bain's long epistle when I bade them good night. Not a word of even second hand news from Zetland which has much disappointed me. . . .

April 21st. – Saw Capt. Benson, he is extremely sick; made enquiries at him concerning the fowls for Mr. Hay. Acknowledged there were a parcel of geese and turkeys on board but that he did not know for whom they were intended; supposed any one to whom they belonged would immediately apply for them as he understood there was a letter accompanying them. There being two letters for Mr. Hay by the brig, rather than lose the chance of getting the fowls, which I saw I should be in some danger of doing unless I could shew some authority to get possession of them, I resolved on opening one which had the appearance of being a Batavia communication, although the hand writing was evidently not that of J. Fea . . . It was a letter from Captain Lee who left this with the brig *Philotas* under his charge, on finding which I shut it again without perusing its contents. There was nothing farther for it therefore but to wait whether any other person came forward to claim them. . . .

April 22nd. – No claimant appearing for the fowls, Capt. Benson has allowed me to send on board for them, though conditionally that if any other person shews hereafter a preferable right Mr. Hay will have to return the whole or a proportionate part of them. There were originally shipt 8 dozen geese and 1 dozen turkeys, and there are now landed only 19 of the former and 7 of the latter. Wrote Mr. Hay in the forenoon . . .

April 23rd. – This being the anniversary of His Majesty King George the Fourth's birth day was noticed as such in the morning by a royal salute from the artillery on the Plain; another took place at midday; and the day was finished by a dinner party on the Government Hill at 7 o'clock which was so ill attended and stupid it scarce merits notice.

Received a letter from Mr. Hay by the *Fazel Currim*, in which he orders an additional supply of clothes and some biscuits. Sent them by a sampan pucat which goes across early in the morning, along with two letters from myself, one containing his Batavia letters and two copies of the last number of the Singapore Chronicle. . . .

April 3rd. [sic] – In the morning on coming to the office, am surprised to find Mr. Read there before me, which unwonted sight may be accounted for by the American brigs making preparation for sailing. . . . We send up on speculation by this brig 30 chests Patna opium of the 2nd Sale, invoiced at $1.550 cts., in the hopes of getting it disposed of before the news of its fall in Calcutta gets wind at Canton, and as the Supercargo of the brig is a speculator in Turkey opium to a considerable amount himself . . . and being too the first vessel that has gone on for that place, there is a probability if there is a market for opium at all it may turn out not a losing concern. But at the same time it is a great risk, as many accidents may occur to detain him on the voyage, and there will be numerous vessels following on his heels. . . .

April 25th. – Sunday. Before breakfast finished a letter I had previously commenced for my Uncle Laurence. Sent John down to Mr. Armstrong's for a cloth jackcoat he is getting made for me, and two drums of a fresh importation of Turkey figs that have been sent up from Batavia consigned to Mr. Read for sale. They were intended for Mr. Hay, in conformity with a request he makes to Mr. Read in a letter from Rhio. The drums, being larger than I had fancied them to be, I returned one. I received the Jackcoat. At midday went down to the office, where I found Mr. Johnston and Mr. Read both busy writing, chiefly for their private correspondents, unless one from Mr. J. to Mr. T. Raffles which I copied in the letter book. Finding nothing to do and disliking to leave the place while they continued in it, took it into my head to write Andrew, and once engaged in so doing, tipped William a letter also. Did not get away till near 4 p.m. Delivered the letters to Dr. Cochrane of the ship *Mary*, who sails in a day or two. Dined at Mr. Read's . . .

WALTER SCOTT DUNCAN
Duncan's Journal
The Straits Times, January 1883

26

1830 & 1833
A Visit to the Rajah

A naturalist and surgeon, George Bennett travelled widely in the East for the purpose of "observations in natural history". In this spirit of scientific enquiry he paid two visits to the "rajah of Johore", also known as Sultan Hussein, who was then living in Singapore at Kampong Glam.

One evening, accompanied by several gentlemen resident in the settlement, I went to pay a visit to the rajah of Johore. During a former visit to this settlement, in 1830, I had an interview with this exalted personage, of whom at that time I penned the following description:-

"Being near the village of Kampong Glam, I observed a poor-looking bungalow, surrounded by high walls, exhibiting effects of age and climate. Over the large gateway which opened into the inclosure surrounding this dwelling were watch-towers. On inquiry, I found this was the residence of the rajah of Johore, who formerly included Singapore in his dominions. The island was purchased of him by the British government, who now allow him an annual pension. He is considered to have been formerly a leader of pirates; and when we saw a brig he was building, it naturally occurred to our minds whether he was about to resort to his old practices. We proposed visiting this personage; and, on arriving at the gateway, were met by a peon, who, after delivering our message to the rajah, requested us to wait a few minutes, until his *Highness* was ready. We did not wait long, for the rajah soon appeared, and took his seat, in lieu of a throne, upon the highest step of those which led to his dwelling. His appearance was remarkable: he appeared a man of about forty years of age – teeth perfect, but quite black, from the custom of chewing the betel constantly.

27

His head was large; and his shaven cranium afforded an interesting phrenological treat. He was deformed; not more than five feet in height, of large body, and short, thick, and deformed legs, scarcely able to support the ponderous trunk. His neck was thick and short, and his head habitually stooped; his face bloated, with the lower lip projecting, and large eyes protruding, one of them having a cataractal appearance. He was dressed in a short pair of cotton drawers, a sarong of cotton cloth came across the shoulders in the form of a scarf, and tarnished, embroidered slippers, and handkerchief around the head, (having the upper part exposed,) after the Malay fashion, completed the attire of this singular creature.

"As much grace and dignity was displayed in our reception as such a figure could show, and chairs were placed by the attendants for our accommodation. He waddled a short distance, and, notwithstanding the exertion was so extraordinary as to cause large drops of perspiration to roll down his face, conferred a great honour upon us by personally accompanying us to see a tank he had just formed for fish, and with a flight of steps, for the convenience of bathing. After viewing this, he returned to his former station, when he reseated himself, with a dignity of look and manner surpassing all description; and we took our departure, after a brief common-place conversation. . . ."

The buildings of his highness and followers were now in some degree improved, being surrounded by a neat chunamed wall, and the entrance was by a gateway of brick, which had been only recently completed. Since my last visit his highness had caused a house to be constructed after the style of the European residents at Singapore, and it was situated exterior to the old boundary of his domain. We were ushered into the new house, the rooms of which were furnished after the English style, with wall-lamps, bookcase, (minus books,) tables, chairs, &c.; ascending to the upper room, chairs were placed for our accommodation, and the punka was caused to be moved to cool our frames. When we were all seated, a yellow painted armed chair was placed at the head of the room, as a regal seat for his highness; his prime minister came to us, and, as we thought, seemed puzzled for what so large a party of Europeans could require an audience.

At last a messenger entered the room, and, squatting down near the minister, whispered something to him, which it seemed was a desire that we should adjourn from this to the old thatched residence of the Tuan rajah. We adjourned, therefore; and, on arriving at the old residence, the rajah, one of the greatest curiosities of the human race perhaps ever seen, waddled, bending with infirmities, and seated his carcase in the aforesaid yellow chair, which had been brought from the other house, and placed in a suitable situation; and there, with his corpulent body completely jammed between the arms of the chair, received us in a most gracious and condescending manner, if such a figure really could look gracious or condescending.

The creature was tame, and both mentally and physically more debilitated than when I last saw him, in 1830: he appeared not even to possess the intelligence of an orang-utan; he was attired in a dirty sarong around his waist, and a loose baju, or jacket, exposing the corpulency of his *delicate* form. A Moorman's cap ornamented a small portion of his cranium; his look was listless, and without any expression: he appeared every moment to be in danger of an attack of apoplexy. The gentlemen who spoke the Malay language, on addressing him, received a grunt, or his language was so unintelligible that his minister was obliged to repeat the answers. All the attendants sat down upon their haunches in his presence, out of respect.

On asking him his age, he replied (or rather his minister for him) by demanding how old we thought he was; we certainly thought he had not yet attained the age of reason. We were afterwards told his age was not exactly known, but it was supposed the creature was fifty. As but little could be made out of this pitiable object of humanity, we released him from what certainly must have been to him a misery, by taking our leave. On viewing the edifices in his enclosure, previous to departing, we found the creature amused himself with building. Besides the new residence and wall, he was erecting a residence and wall for himself, neat and extensive in construction, and in something of a Chinese style of architecture. This building was certainly wanting, for the old thatched palace near it seemed ready to fall about his ears.

GEORGE BENNETT
Wanderings in New South Wales,
Batavia, Pedir Coast, Singapore
and China **(1834)**

1833–34

Occupations

George Windsor Earl was a trader and travel writer who later turned to law and Government service. At the time of this extract Earl was in his late twenties and trading extensively in the region, using Singapore as his base. In this way he came to know Singapore well.

An early walk through Campong Glam will serve to give a stranger a good idea of the habits and occupations of the different classes. Near the residence of the Sultan he will meet with Malays, lounging about near the doors of their houses, chewing betel, with their sarongs, which usually hang loosely about the waist, wrapped round the body to shelter the wearer from the cool morning breeze. The main street, however, will have a very different appearance. There Chinese mechanics will be busily employed forging ironwork, making furniture, or building boats; and the level green near the sea will be occupied by Bugis, who have landed from their prahus to mend their sails, or to twist rope and cables from the materials which they have brought with them. In a portion of the back part of the campong, natives of Sambawa, a far distant island to the eastward of Java, will be found chopping young trees into billets for fire-wood, and making hurdles for fencing; and in another, Bengali washermen hanging out clothes to dry, and dairymen of the same nation milking their cows to supply the breakfast tables of the Europeans. On the roads Klings will occasionally be encountered conducting tumbrils drawn by buffaloes cased in mud and dirt; the creaking of the wheels almost drowning the voice of the driver as he bawls to the animals, in his harsh and discordant jargon. Each nation, indeed, is found pursuing avocations which best accord with its tastes and habits. . . .

From five thousand to eight thousand emigrants arrive annually from China, of whom only forty or fifty are females. About one-

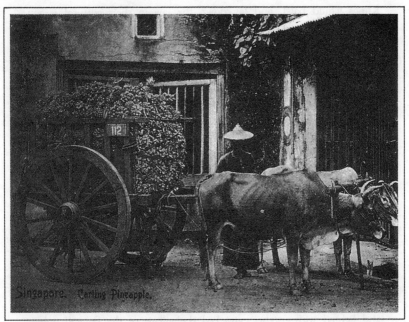

CARTING PINEAPPLE

eighth of these people remain at Singapore, and the others scatter themselves over the Archipelago. . . .

The landing of the emigrants from the junks forms a very interesting sight, and if I happened to be in the town at the arrival of a large junk, I generally stationed myself near the landing-place to watch their proceedings. They usually came on shore in large cargo-boats, each carrying from fifty to sixty persons, scarcely any space being left for the rowers. As the boat approached the landing-place, which was always on those occasions crowded with Chinese, the emigrants would cast anxious glances among them, and a ray of delight would occasionally brighten the countenance of one of the "high aspirants," on recognizing the face of a relative or friend, on whose favourable report he had probably decided on leaving his country. The boat was always anchored a short distance from the landing-place, and a squabble would immediately commence between the Kling boatmen and the Chinese passengers, many of the latter being unprovided with the few halfpence required to pay their passage from the vessel. The

Klings would bawl, and lay down the law in their guttural jargon, and the Chinese would remonstrate in scarcely less barbarous Fokeen, each being totally unintelligible to the other. After some delay the boat would be pushed in for the shore, and the emigrants, taking up their sleeping mats and small bundles, which formed all their worldly wealth, would proceed to the abodes of their friends, or scatter themselves over the town in search of lodgings. . . .

The majority of the emigrants embark in China without sufficient money to pay their passage to Singapore, and these defaulters remain in the vessel until they are redeemed by their friends, who pay the amount; or by strangers engaging their services for a stipulated period, and paying their passage money as an advance of wages. The mechanics soon acquire capital, as they always work hard on their first arrival; but many, finding that money can be easily obtained, indulge in gambling and opium-smoking, becoming eventually as dissolute as they were previously industrious. . . .

The houses in the outskirts of the town are often attacked by bands of Chinese robbers from the interior, but fortunately they are such arrant cowards that they retreat on the slightest opposition. One fine night during my stay, a body of about fifty, armed with spears and lighted with torches, attacked the village of the Bengali dobies. The dobies fled, and the Chinese seized upon the linen, clean and dirty, and hastened back towards their fastnesses, bearing away a fair proportion of the wardrobes of the European ladies and gentlemen. Although the cowardly washermen thought of nothing save flight, the robbers did not retreat unmolested, for a gentleman who resided on the outskirts of the town having witnessed their descent, mustered two or three Malays, armed with a couple of fowling-pieces, and laid wait near the road-side for their return. As the robbers passed, triumphing in the idea of carrying away so much valuable booty, of shirts and petticoats, the little party fired, and brought down two of them, on which the remainder took to flight, utterly regardless of the fate of their comrades. The assailants pursued, and the robbers, to escape as they supposed impending destruction, dropped their bundles, so that their line of retreat was pointed out next morning by the wearing apparel scattered on the road, which was collected and returned to the rightful owners. . . .

The two Malay chiefs residing in the settlement are both *pensionnaires* of the East-India Company. One is the Sultan of Johore, a neighbouring state on the Peninsula, by whom Singapore and the islands near the coast were ceded to the British; and the other is the Tumung-gung, a petty chief, nominally a tributary to the Sultan, who was found in possession of the country about Singapore. . . .

The Tumung-gung is a young man, and like most of the nobles, remarkable, even among the Malays, for his depravity. Although a *pensionnaire* of the Company to the annual amount of four thousand five hundred dollars, he is strongly suspected of encouraging the pirates, who, for years have been murdering and plundering the native traders almost within sight of the harbour; and, if not personally engaged in piratical pursuits, it is well known that many of those in his confidence are absent for considerable periods under very suspicious circumstances. The Tumung-gung resides in a village exclusively inhabited by Malays, situated in a small cove about a mile and a half to the westward of the town, from which it is entirely concealed by the intervening hills.

The Malay pirates absolutely swarm in the neighbourhood of Singapore, the numerous islands in the vicinity, the intersecting channels of which are known only to themselves, affording them a snug retreat, whence they can pounce upon the defenceless native traders, and drag them into their lairs to plunder them at their leisure. Square-rigged vessels are generally allowed to pass unmolested, for the pirates, who are as cowardly as they are cruel, rarely attack craft of this description, unless they have received authentic information from their spies at Singapore that they may be taken with facility.

The system of piracy is perfect in its nature, more so even than that which formerly obtained among the Buccaneers of America. A petty chief of one of the Malay states, who has either been ruined by gambling, or is desirous to improve his fortune, collects under his banner as many restless spirits as he can muster, and sails for one of the most retired islands in the neighbourhood of Singapore. Here he erects a village as a depôt for slaves and plunder, and then lies in wait with his armed prahus, near the frequented waters, for the native traders passing to and from the British settlement. Should the chief be eminently successful, he soon gains a large accession to his force, and his village increases to a small town, while his fleet of prahus becomes sufficiently numerous to be subdivided into several squadrons, which cruise in the various straits and channels.

The pirates generally sail in fleets of from three to twenty prahus. These are armed with guns, large and small, and each prahu carries from fifteen to forty men. The vessels which they succeed in capturing are brought to the settlement, where they are plundered and afterwards burnt; and the goods are taken for sale to Singapore or New Harbour, in prahus of their own, which are fitted up to resemble traders. The unfortunate natives who compose the crews of the captured prahus, are carried to Lingin, or to the opposite coast of Sumatra, where they are sold to the Malays, to cultivate the pepper plantations in the interior.

GEORGE WINDSOR EARL
The Eastern Seas (1837)

Scorpions in the Cabin

Howard Malcolm, an American missionary, spent a month in Singapore while on an inspection tour of the missions in the region. He begins this extract by describing the conditions on board a small coasting vessel such as many Singapore visitors must have experienced on their journey.

You find, on getting aboard, a cabin five or six feet square, and are fortunate if in it you can stand erect, and still more so if it have a port-hole, or any ventilation, except through the scuttle, by which you enter. Here you eat with the captain, or perhaps off of a stinking hen-coop on deck. There can be no awning on deck, because it would be in the way of the boom; so that you stay below, while the sun blazes on the plank over your head, and keeps the thermometer in the cabin about blood heat. Your mattress is laid on a locker at night, and rolled up in the day. Perhaps you may be able to swing it. The seams on deck, neglected and parched up, during a six months' dry season, let the salt water on you in rapid drops, when the decks are washed. If it be rainy season, your confinement below is scarcely less unpleasant. Trunks and small stores must occupy the margin of the cabin, or be stowed where you cannot come at them. If you attempt to write, three times a day you must huddle together your papers, that the trunk or table may be spread for meals; or if you eat on deck, and so have uninterrupted use of the table, the heat and motion make study difficult. Your cooking is by no means scientific. The fowls, sometimes without the privilege of a coop, and lying on the deck tied by the legs, "get no better very fast." The smallness of the vessel makes her toss about most uncomfortably, when a larger vessel would be quite still; so that, if you take anything out of its place, it must be "chocked" again with care, or it will "fetch way." As to walking the deck, there is hardly room to turn; and if there be, you must have either the sun or dew upon you. But your worst time is at night. Several must sleep in the tiny cabin; and the heavy, damp air, coming down the gangway, gives you rheumatism, without producing ventilation. You perspire at every pore, till nature is exhausted, and you sleep, from very inanity.

There are other disagreeables, which, though worse, are happily not quite so common. Some of the captains have no means of ascertaining latitude, and still fewer their longitude. Sometimes there is no chart on board. The cables, anchors, and general inventory, are apt to be poor. Vessels in the habit of carrying rice, timber, stick-lac, &c., have always mice, cockroaches, centipedes, scorpions, and ants, in great abundance. In one of my voyages, I killed nearly thirty scorpions in the cabin, and in another, eight or ten centipedes. Thrice, on taking out of my trunk a clean shirt, I found a centipede in its folds. Large, winged cockroaches infest all Indian vessels; but in some they creep about in every direction, day and night. I had one full specimen of this. Such crowds lighted upon the dinner-table, that we could hardly tell meat from potatoes. To drive them away and eat at the same time was impossible, for they would keep off of a dish no longer than it was agitated. The captain and I just dined patiently, each contenting himself with being able to keep them out of his own plate. At night, they swarmed in thousands on the boards and on the bed, eating our fingers and toes to the quick. A hundred oranges, tied up in a bag, had not been on board thirty-six hours, before it was found that these cormorants had left nothing but the skin. It was a bag full of hollow globes! . . .

These things ought not, perhaps, in strictness, to be called hardships, but they are inconveniences, which I found tended rapidly to make me old, and convince me that voyages of this sort cannot be a wise resort for invalid missionaries.

In going through one part of the town, during business hours, one feels himself to be in a Chinese city. Almost every respectable native he sees is Chinese; almost every shop, ware-room, and trade, is carried on by the Chinese; the hucksters, coolies, travelling cooks, and cries common in a great city, are Chinese. In fact, we may almost call Singapore itself a Chinese city; inasmuch as the bulk of the inhabitants are Chinese, and nearly all the wealth and influence, next to the British, is in their hands. A large part of the Klings and Bengalese are ostlers, servants, washermen, &c., to Europeans; and the Malays

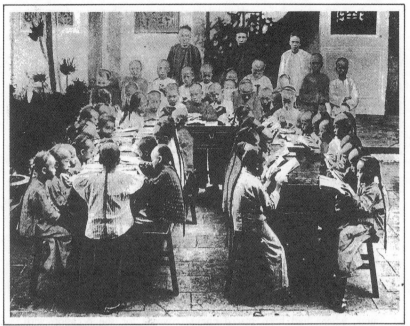

CHINESE BOY'S SCHOOL

and Bugis occupy portions of the city by themselves. . . .

A Chinese population of so many thousands, gave me many opportunities of observing the manners of this singular people. One of these was a wedding, to which I had the pleasure of being invited, through the kind offices of Mr. Ballistier, our American consul, to whom I was much indebted in other respects. As I had no hope of such an opportunity in China, I gladly availed myself of this. The family of the bride being wealthy, the room containing the family altar was decorated both with costliness and taste. The *"Jos"* was delineated in a large picture surrounded by ornamental paper-hangings. Huge wax candles, delicate tapers, and suspended lamps, of elegantly painted glass, shed round their formal light, though it was broad day. On the altar, or table, before the idol, were trays of silver and rich porcelain, filled with offerings of sweetmeats and flowers, while burning sandal-wood and agillocha, diffused a pleasing fragrance.

After the elders had performed their devotions, the bride came slowly in, supported by attendants, and went through tedious gestures,

37

and genuflections before the idol, without raising her eyes from the ground, or speaking. Her robe was both gorgeous and graceful, covering her, in loose folds, so completely that neither her feet nor hands could be seen. Beside the numerous ornaments and jewels which bound up her profuse hair, she wore several heavy necklaces of sparkling jewels, apparently artificial. When she had finished, an elder placed on her head a thick veil, and she returned to her apartment. We now waited for the bridegroom, who "tarried" a little, and the interval was enlivened by tea, sweetmeats, betel-nut, &c. Three bands of music, European, Malay, and Javanese, sent sounds of gladness through the halls and corridors; the friends passed about with smiles and greetings; the children, in their gay apparel, danced joyously, they knew not why; – all was natural and pleasing, but the slow and extravagant movements of a Javanese dancing-girl, who, in a corner of the porch, earned her pay, little regarded.

At length it was heralded, "the bridegroom cometh," and immediately many "went forth to meet him." He came with friends and a priest, preceded by another band of music. His devotions before the Jos, were much sooner and more slightly done than those of the lady; and he sat down with the priest, and a friend or two, in front of the altar, where had been placed chairs, covered for the occasion with loose drapery of embroidered velvet. Refreshments were handed, till a movement from within announced the approach of the bride; and all eyes were turned to meet her. She advanced very slowly to the centre, veiled, as when she retired, and, after a few gestures by each toward the other, the happy pair sat down together, her face still invisible. Refreshments again entered, and each partook, but with evident agitation and constraint. Presently, she retired to her chamber, followed by the bridegroom; and most of the guests dispersed; but we were permitted, with some particular friends, to enter with them. It was doubtless a handsome room in Chinese estimation, but its decorations would scarcely please a Western eye. The bedstead resembled a latticed arbor; and from the roof within was suspended a beautiful lamp of chased silver, burning with a feeble light. Standing in the middle of the room, they renewed their bowing, and passing from side to side, with a gravity and tediousness almost ludicrous, till he finished the ceremony by approaching and lifting the veil from her head. We were told that till then he had never seen her! She blushed, and sat without raising her eyes; but, alas for the romance of the thing – she was ugly! A leisurely repast followed, shared by themselves

38

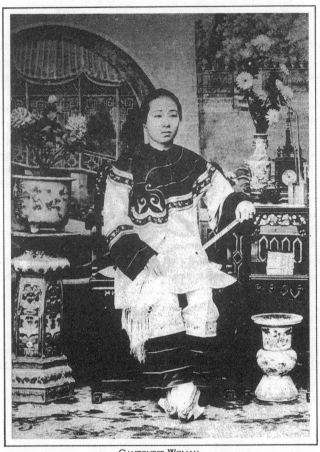

CANTONESE WOMAN

alone; and probably forming the ratifying feature of the solemnity, as in Burmah. Fifty dishes or more were before them, a few of which they tasted with silver forks; but of course the occasion was too ethereal to be substantiated by veritable eating and drinking. When they rose from the table, the bridegroom, aided by his servant, removed his outer robe, which had been worn as a dress of ceremony, and threw it on the bed, as if marking it for his own. Then, advancing respectfully to the bride, her attendant raised the folds of her dress, and he unclasped the cincture of the garment beneath. This act, so gentle, delicate, and significant, closed the ceremonial. He then returned to his own house till evening, and every guest retired – a capital system, allowing the bride some repose, after the trying and tiresome ceremonies she had performed. This was about four o'clock. In the evening, a sumptuous entertainment was given to the friends of both parties; after which the bridegroom remained, as a son at home.

More refined deportment cannot be, than was exhibited by all parties on this occasion. The guests were not all at one table, nor even in one room; but many tables were spread, each accommodating five or six persons, and all diverse in their viands. Servants were numerous, the silver and porcelain handsome, the deportment of the guests unexceptionable, and sobriety universal. Every thing testified the high claim of the Chinese to the character of a civilized people.

I readily accepted an invitation, a few evenings afterward, to an entertainment at the same house. Order, delicacy, abundance, and elegance, reigned throughout. Of course many of the dishes were new to me, but there were many also, in exact English style. Among the novelties, I tried sharks' fins, birds' nests, fish-maws, and Biche-de-mer. I think an unprejudiced taste would pronounce them good; but only that of a Chinese would consider them delicacies.

HOWARD MALCOLM
Travels in South-Eastern Asia,
embracing Hindustan, Malaya, Siam,
and China (1839)

c. 1844

For Recovery of Health

Dr. James Thomas Oxley was first posted to Singapore in 1830, and in 1844 was appointed Senior Surgeon for the Straits Settlements. Although it has been said that he showed more interest in his nutmeg plantations than in his official medical duties, his advice to invalids seeking convalescence in Singapore was no doubt read with respect.

Those who only purpose making the trip for the benefit of the voyage and a few days stay at Singapore can be tolerably well accomodated, at two respectable Hotels; where if they do not obtain luxuries they can at all events get good wholesome necessaries, for such sojourners Hotel accomodation is sufficient, but for individuals or families who wish to avoid some of the hottest months in Calcutta by a more continued residence here it will be preferable to rent a House. These are generally procurable of a sufficiently commodious description, in eligible situations for from 30 to 40 Dollars a month, they can be readily furnished from the shops of the Chinese carpenters at trifling expense, probably realizing by auction on the departure of the owner within 10 or 15 per cent of original cost. Good fish and poultry are abundant. Fowls full grown are to be had at about $3 the dozen, Turkeys $2 per pair, Ducks $3½ per dozen, Geese $1 each, Mutton is procurable two or three times a week of excellent quality, an hind quarter costs $3, Beef is tough, lean and generally unfit for use except as soup-meat . . . I would recommend persons leaving Calcutta to bring all their household servants with them, those they will find here are of the very worst description, and exorbitant in their demand for wages, Chinese are to be procured for out door work, but are not safe to be trusted where there is temptation, particularly by strangers, when good they are about the best class of household servants, but when bad they are clever and dangerous rogues. There are numbers of palankeen carriages for hire in the Bazaar,

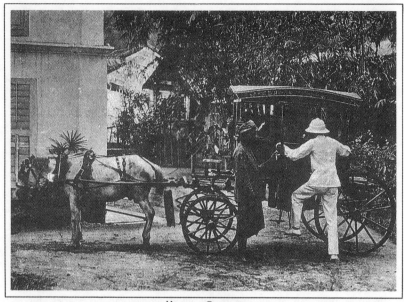

HACKNEY CARRIAGE

but they are dirty, unsightly vehicles and for the most part quite unfit for a Lady's use. The hire per month is about 25 Dollars for one of the best, so that persons intending to make this their place of residence for some months had better bring with them a Light Pony Phaeton if they wish to be comfortable, good Ponies are generally procurable for from 50 to $100 each. If the visitor be particular about his wines he had better lay in a stock at Calcutta, those procurable here are always inferior. Europe articles such as Hams, Jams and all Oilman's stores are generally abundant and reasonable. The visitor must not expect to find many external resources here, the Community being composed of working busy people, they have no time to throw away upon idlers, who left to themselves are apt to complain of neglect, this is not altogether fair or reasonable, a man's business must always be paramount to the gratification of cultivating new acquaintances. The roads are pretty good and the drives about Town numerous, the longest Road from Town is about 12 miles. Pleasant little excursions may be made to neighbouring Islands or round the Island of Singapore itself, a trip that must afford full gratification to the lover of the picturesque, the waving outline of the Island with its pretty little coves, and occasional sandy Beach, the varying tints of foliage from the small hills which stud the Island being placed at different planes of elevation and covered with various sorts of Trees, the jutting headlands which on the northern side project so far as to give the voyager the idea of sailing through a series of beautiful Lakes, so completely do you appearto be shut in by them, the smooth clear water, all contribute to form a scene calculated to soothe the irritability of the invalid and gratify the admirer of nature's loveliness. So far the Invalid can enjoy the best exercises for the recovery of health, in occasional boating, or riding and driving in the open air during the cool mornings and evenings which he can remain out with perfect safety until 7 o'clock unless on some particularly hot morning. May and June are less agreeable than the rest of the year from the prevalence of the southerly winds and it is rather remarkable that the stronger these winds blow the more enervating they are, strangers are very apt to sit in this wind and call it a fine breeze, old Residents cannot do so with impunity, on the contrary they carefully avoid its influence. I would strongly advise all who are desirous of keeping their health to carefully exclude it, even at the expense of temporary heat and discomfort. There are no public amusements or even Library in the place and the only lion is the Chinese temple at Teluk Ayer, which as a specimen of Chinese taste and rich carving is not unworthy of a visit. Although the heat during the day is frequently oppressive the nights are always sufficiently cool to allow of refreshing sleep and this alone to an invalid is of vast importance and is perhaps upon the whole the greatest avantage to be derived by a change from continental India to the Straits.

DR. J.T. OXLEY
"Advice to Invalids Resorting to Singapore"
Journal of the Indian Archipelago
and Eastern Asia, **Vol. V, April 1851**
Ed. J.R. Logan

Shooting the Stag

For half a century Douglas Hamilton (later General Hamilton) kept a journal of his experiences, from which comes this account of sporting life in Singapore. At the time, Hamilton was a twenty-eight-year-old Captain in the Madras Army and his regiment had been posted for duty in Singapore.

Singapore with its valleys, plains, grand trees and undulating hills, is very beautiful. In 1846 a great portion of the settlement was covered with jungle so dense that it was almost impenetrable and sport was hopeless. There were some deer, muntjack or barking deer, and wild hog on the island, and we managed after many a blank day, to kill a few of these. I was fortunate in shooting the only stag of any size that had been killed on the island for a long time, and the advantage of not wearing any conspicuous colour when out after game was very manifest on this occasion. We were posted by the side of the high road where the forest had been cleared and a scrub jungle had grown up. I saw the stag suddenly appear on some rising ground above the road and deliberately take his bearings. Now as all my companions had something white about them which made them very conspicuous, and I had nothing of the kind visible, he came straight down to where I was standing, and on his coming within shot got the contents of both my barrels which turned him back severely wounded, and he fell dead after proceeding a short distance; a fine beast, 13 hands at the shoulder with small but very thick antlers. They tell me that the deer on the island never have very large antlers. My sporting friends after this event, took great pains to hide every scrap of white in their dress, but no more stags came to be shot. There was said to be a great number of tigers on the island and some hundreds of Chinamen were reported to be killed each year by them, but as the Chinamen belonged to secret societies who were in perpetual feud and always ready to kill each other, I am afraid many a murder has been falsely attributed to the "gentleman in stripes." In respect to this, I was told rather an amusing story of a very knowing Chinaman. The stems of the large cable-like creepers that twine about the forest trees like huge snakes, are valuable on account of their variety of colour and beauty of grain, for wood veneering; the above mentioned individual having found a spot where these valuable creepers abounded and fearing that others might reap the harvest, adopted an ingenious plan to keep them away; he carefully carved a tiger's foot in wood and stamped the impression in every direction leading to this piece of jungle; after a time news was brought in by another wood cutter of these numerous tracks; on first visiting the ground there appeared to be little doubt as to its being much frequented by a tiger, but on carefully inspecting the foot prints, it was discovered that they were *all made by one foot.*

I offered large rewards to get a shot at a tiger, but though I often sat up for one I never once had a chance. There was however some very fair snipe shooting to be got in the cultivated grounds. . . .

One of my chief amusements at Singapore was "paddling my own canoe" amongst the lovely islands and looking down into the coral covered depths below, which on a calm day seemed like a fairy forest, the coral having a most tree-like appearance and of every variety of tint from deep red to the most delicate green. Fish of all sizes and colours were swimming about in every direction far down in these charming water woods. So clear is the sea that the Malays in their sanpans, a very light kind of canoe, chase and spear the seer fish, which here takes the place of salmon, only the flesh is white instead of pink. It is a fast swimmer, quite as large as the salmon and excellent eating. Two Malays, one in the bow and the other in the stern of the canoe, paddle out in search of the fish and on finding a shoal give chase; the man at the bow, besides his paddle, has a long three pronged bamboo spear, like an eel spear, and wears a large shade over his eyes to assist him in seeing into the depths below. The pace they go and the turns and doubles they make is very exciting, and the excitement increases when the man at the bow stands up and with the spear balancing above his head prepares to strike – now he is going to throw! No! he calmly puts the spear down and paddles with all his might at one time passing close to you, then dashing off far away, suddenly doubling back again — now he is up once more, and the spear quivers in his hand. Now! Now! No, he calmly lays down the spear again and is paddling away as hard as ever. This sometimes is repeated over and over again and my patience has been sorely tried when looking on, the calm unexcited bearing of the spearman making it still more provoking. At last the spear is thrown and with such unerring aim that I have never to my recollection seen a failure. The spear is heavily weighted at the base so that it throws up the fish, and being made fast to the boat by a line is easily hauled in. I have seen fish of between 20 and 30 lbs. captured in this way. It is also interesting to watch the ospreys or fishing eagles, of which there were numbers, soaring high above and dropping like a bullet into the sea, rising again with a good sized fish in their talons.

GENERAL DOUGLAS HAMILTON
Records of Sport in Southern India
also including notes on Singapore,
Java and Labuan (1892)

1848

Attacked by a Tiger

As a British naval captain Henry Keppel was actively involved in anti-piracy operations in the region, but he is best remembered for championing the development of the New Harbour in Singapore (renamed Keppel Harbour in 1900). Later to become Admiral and Sir Henry, he first visited Singapore in 1833 and returned many times during the next seventy years. Throughout his lifetime tigers remained a real problem in Singapore.

During our stay at Sincapore, the body of a large tiger was brought in by some Malays (a not unusual occurrence), to enable them to receive the reward given by Government. The Malays stated that, when they found this monster in a hole which had been dug to catch him, they threw quick lime into his eyes; and the unfortunate beast, while suffering intense agony from this cruel appliance, drowned himself in some water which was at the bottom of the pit, though not more than a foot deep.

The annual loss of human life from tigers, chiefly among the Chinese settlers, is perfectly fearful, averaging no fewer than 360, or one per diem. Great exertions are still making for the destruction of these animals, which is effected by pitfalls, cages baited with a dog, goat, monkey, or other restless animal, and by sundry cunning contrivances. Not many years ago the existence of a tiger in the island was disbelieved; and they must have been very scarce indeed, for even the natives did not know of any. It is the opinion of Dr. Oxley (no mean authority at Sincapore), that one may have been accidentally carried by the tide across the narrow straits which separate the island from the main land, and another may have instinctively followed: finding abundance of food they have multiplied. This is a more rational mode of accounting for their being here, than to suppose that they chased their prey over; as it is contrary to the nature of the beast to follow in

47

pursuit, after the first attempt proves unsuccessful. Now, at Sincapore, as in the days of Alfred with the wolves in England, it is necessary to offer a reward for their destruction.

One of the most recent victims was the son of the headman at the village of Passier Rice, who, having gone into the jungle immediately at the back of his father's house, for the purpose of cutting wood, was attacked by a tiger. The father, hearing his cries, rushed out just in time to grasp his son's legs, as the brute was dragging him into the jungle. The father pulled and the tiger growled ferociously, and it was only on several persons coming up and assailing him, that the monster was persuaded to quit his prey; but the unfortunate young man was dead! I could enumerate many instances of the daring exploits of these brutes, but one or two will be sufficient to convince the reader of the ferocious nature of their attacks, and their peculiar relish for human flesh, which, when once tasted, is preferred by them to any other.

The district of Siranjong appears to be their favourite prowling-ground. In April, last year, one of them put to flight a party of Malays who were at work in that neighbourhood. Before they could get clear of the jungle, the tiger – a well-known brute, advanced in years, and remarkable from having large white spots – sprang upon one of them, selecting, of course, the fattest. When the first shock of their fright was over, they turned on the tiger, and, pursuing him with their parongs (short swords), made him drop his prey, but not until the poor man was in the agonies of death. The same tiger, however, determined not to be disappointed of his meal, that night carried off a Chinaman at a short distance from the scene of his morning's exploits. In the course of the following month, at the same place, two Chinamen employed in sawing timber were carried off. On the last occasion, the comrades of the victim, hearing his shrieks, bravely rushed out in a body to his assistance, as the tiger was dragging him towards the jungle; but, instead of dropping his prey and skulking off as he ought to have done, the brute, greatly to their dismay, faced about and stood growling over the body in a most ferocious manner; and it was not until he had received a shower of sticks and stones that he moved off.

The water-buffalo is an animal much in use at Sincapore for purposes of draught. It is a dull, heavy-looking animal – slow at work, and I think disgusting in appearance; but remarkable for sagacity and attachment to its native keepers. It has, however, a particular antipathy to a European, and will immediately detect him in a crowd. Its dislike to, and its courage in attacking, the tiger is well known all over India.

Not long ago, as a Malayan boy, who was employed by his parents in herding some water-buffaloes, was driving his charge home by the borders of the jungle, a tiger made a sudden spring, and, seizing the lad by the thigh, was dragging him off, when two old bull buffaloes, hearing the shriek of distress from the well-known voice of their little attendant, turned round and charged with their usual rapidity. The tiger, thus closely pressed, was obliged to drop his prey, to defend himself. While one buffalo fought and successfully drove the tiger away, the other kept guard over the wounded boy. Later in the evening, when the anxious father, alarmed, came out with attendants to seek his child, he found that the whole herd, with the exception of the two old buffaloes, had dispersed themselves to feed, but that *they* were still there – one standing over the bleeding body of their little friend, while the other kept watch on the edge of the jungle for the return of the tiger.

There is a procession and much parade in bringing these tigers to the Government office. They are made to look as fierce as .possible, propped up in a standing position by pieces of bamboo, the mouth open, and tail on end.

The Governor kindly presented me with this fallen monarch of the jungle, and I was astonished at the number of native volunteers for the service of denuding him of his skin, the only part I coveted, while they demanded the carcase for their trouble. But I found afterwards that they made a large profit by retailing the flesh, a belief being entertained by this people that the eating of it is not only a sovereign remedy for all diseases, but that it imparts to him who eats it the sagacity as well as the courage of the animal. A friend of mine belonging to the 21st regiment, M.N.I., who was slowly recovering from an attack of fever, finding some difficulty in masticating the food before him, questioned his servant as to the cause, when he discovered that the fellow had purchased a small piece of my tiger, which he had clandestinely introduced into his master's currie. When my friend got well, young Zaddie firmly believed that his remedy had effected the cure.

CAPT^{n.} THE HON. HENRY KEPPEL, R.N.
*A Visit to the Indian Archipelago
in H.M. Ship Mæander* (1852)

1851

A Cottage in the Jungle

Ida Pfeiffer, an Austrian widow from Vienna, wrote of herself: "I am a most simple and unpretending person, and can claim as a writer no merit whatever, beyond that of describing truly and without exaggeration what I have seen and experienced." After Singapore, Mrs. Pfeiffer went on to explore Sarawak and the Dutch East Indies. She was fifty-four.

The distance from the entrance of the Strait of Sunda to Singapore is not more than seven degrees, but, having to contend with contrary winds and calms, we took fourteen days to it, crossing the equator full half-a-dozen times, and during several nights coming to anchor. The heat was almost intolerable. It rose in the shade to 92½° Fahr.; but the time nevertheless passed pretty quickly. The captain was an educated man, and moreover could play the flute. The natives of the places we passed occasionally paid us visits, bringing with them poultry and fruit, which they exchanged for handkerchiefs, little looking-glasses, or money; and thus kept our table well provided; and the variety of the ever-changing scenery of the shore amused me so much, that I am afraid I can hardly claim any merit for having borne this fourteen days' passage with perfect patience.

We had nevertheless some disagreeable incidents. One morning a sailor, while employed in furling a sail, fell overboard; and on the very same day the same accident happened to the chief mate, while he was taking soundings. Fortunately there was little or no wind, and both were saved.

One night we were threatened with a still more unpleasant adventure. We were lying at anchor, and since these seas are frequently infested by pirates, the captain had given strict orders to have a vigilant watch kept. We went to bed, but had scarcely got to sleep, when we were startled by the cry from deck, "Two boats in sight from the land!"

Everybody sprang up in a moment. Muskets, ammunition, pistols, and sabres were quickly brought on deck, and distributed among the crew; our two six-pounders, the only guns we carried, were loaded; and in this grand attitude we awaited the foe. But after all, the two boats never came near us, and we were subsequently told that these pirates scarcely ever do attack European ships.

We reached Singapore on the 16th of November, after a fifty-four days' voyage from the Cape, and I was received by the Behn family with the same kindness as when, four years previously, I visited the place for the first time.

In Singapore itself I found nothing altered, but a magnificent lighthouse had been built during that time, about twenty miles off the island, on a rock in the sea, where there is so tremendous a surf that the guardians of the lighthouse are kept furnished with fresh water and provisions for six months. The tower took eighteen months to build, and is constructed of masses of granite brought from the neighbouring island of Urbin.

It happened, fortunately for me, that a cottage, built just before my arrival, by some families in the country for the sake of enjoying from time to time a better air, just then stood empty; and as Mr. Behn knew that he could afford me no greater pleasure than that of giving me an opportunity of passing a few days in the midst of the jungle, and enjoying to my heart's content the scenery, and the amusement of searching for insects, &c., he placed this cottage at my disposal, and also a boat with five rowers, that I might be able to visit all the little islands around. These five men, who were Malays, used to come every morning to know whether I wanted the boat, and if I did not, they used to attend me in my rambles through the jungle, help me to find insects, &c., and also serve as my protectors against the numerous tigers that swim hither from Malacca across the narrow arm of the sea that divides the peninsula from Singapore. . . .

All the horrible stories I was told, however, did not prevent my finding the greatest delight in roaming from morning till evening in these most beautiful woods. My five brown companions were armed with muskets and long and short knives, and from time to time beat the bushes and trees, and uttered precautionary yells, in order to drive away any bad company they might conceal; but I did not feel at all afraid, for I was busy with the beautiful objects that presented themselves to my observation at every step. Here merry little monkeys were springing from bough to bough, there brightly plumed birds flew suddenly out; plants that seemed to have their roots in the trunks of the trees, twined their flowers and blossoms among the branches or peeped out from the thick foliage; and then again the trees themselves excited my admiration by their size, their height, and their wonderful forms. Never shall I forget the happy days I passed in that Singapore jungle, and I herewith send Mr. Behn from afar my acknowledgments for them.

We saw traces of tigers every day; we found the marks of their claws imprinted in the sand or soft earth; and one day at noon, one of these unwelcome guests came quite near to our cottage, and fetched himself a dog, which he devoured quite at his leisure only a few hundred steps off. One night, too, I was startled from my sleep by a noise in the gallery near my bedroom. I did not think the sound I heard proceeded from a fourfooted animal; but as I was situated, I should have thought biped visitors no less formidable; for at no great distance from the place where I was, there was a sort of government station, where from twenty to thirty criminals were kept, and employed in felling timber. They, in all probability, knew very well that my guards slept in a distant hut, that I was quite alone in the cottage, and that the doors were not, and could not be, locked. I took the precaution, indeed, to have always a large knife near me; but that would most likely have availed me but little, had I really tried to make use of it. I thought it best, however, to put a bold face upon the matter, and cried out in a loud voice, "Who's there?"

I received for an answer that a tiger had been seen, and that they were in pursuit of him — which was perfectly possible; but I did not hear a single shot fired, and the silence of the night was not further disturbed.

IDA PFEIFFER
A Lady's Second Journey Round the World (1855)

For Change of Air

"A Bengal Civilian" – actually Charles W. Kinloch – visited Singapore while on a sea voyage prescribed by his doctors. His view of the place was certainly liverish.

There are several hotels in Singapore, the best of which is the London Hotel, kept by Mr. Du Trouquoy, a native of Jersey; but even in this establishment, there is great room for improvement. The hotel consists of two upper roomed buildings, one of which is styled the Family Hotel. Neither house is comfortable; and the bath room accommodation is especially defective, the whole of the baths being public, and situated in a range of buildings altogether distinct from the hotel. Under the very windows of both hotels is a long tiled building, called a bowling alley. This pandemonium is lit up every night, and is filled with the townspeople and others, who play at bowls and drink brandy and water until a late hour of the night. The alley, as it is called, is very profitable to the proprietor; but it is a great nuisance to the inmates of the hotel. Both hotels face the sea, and command an excellent view of the shipping. But the houses on the beach are not considered the healthiest, and the residents at night time make a practice of closing their venetians in order to exclude the sea breeze, which they consider to be very injurious to health, especially during the prevalence of the southwest monsoon.

Considering the exorbitant prices of even the commonest necessaries of life, the hotel charges cannot be considered high. The charge for a single person breakfasting and dining at the public table being one dollar and a half diem. The charge for families and parties occupying a private sitting room are proportionately higher. The only really objectionable charge in our bill was that for a bath, for which the proprietor asks half a dollar a day, a demand that is most unreasonable, seeing that water is abundant, and close at hand. . . .

There are no places of public resort or amusement at Singapore, neither is there any society. The merchants, who form by far the largest section of the community, seem to look upon money making as the chief end and object of their lives, and their topics of conversation rarely extend to any other subject than that of nutmegs or the last price current. . . .

The Indian visitor will very soon get tired of Singapore, for, setting aside the want of society and the absence of public amusement, the climate is too hot, and too depressing, to render a residence in this island agreeable beyond a period of a few weeks. The average temperature in the town, in a cool house during the southwest monsoon, is 81°. In such a climate, the invalid cannot expect to gain strength, and he may consider himself fortunate if he does not lose ground. To those who have resided for a number of years in the damp atmosphere of Bengal, the climate of the Straits may perhaps be suitable, and, to a certain extent, beneficial; but we should never recommend any of our friends who have lived long in the dry climate of the northwest, to come to Singapore for change of air. . . .

Housekeeping at Singapore is expensive and troublesome, and we would advise the Indian visitor, whether married or unmarried, to take rooms at the hotel, rather than attempt to keep house for himself. Considering the large European society resident at Singapore, there seems no reason why supplies of every kind should not be as abundant there as in Calcutta, but, strange to say, no good beef or mutton is to be had on the island; a small, skinny, sickly looking animal, dignified by the name of a Bengal grain fed sheep, is slaughtered twice a week for the benefit of those who cannot dispense with their mutton chop, and is sold at a fixed price of two and a half dollars a joint. There is always a good supply, however, of good fish in the market, and with that and Chinese pork, the residents are content, but our Indian stomach was not so easily satisfied and we frequently yearned for the . . . beef and grain fed mutton of our Bengal provinces . . .

Amongst the fruits of the Straits, the mangustin has always been deemed pre-eminent, nor do we ever remember to have heard the slightest difference in opinion in regard to the merits of this justly esteemed fruit. We have eaten the very best specimens of the mangustin during our residence here, but much as we approve of the exquisite delicacy and flavour of the fruit, still it has failed to come up to our expectations; and we should not hesitate to accord both to the Bombay mangoe, and to the pine apple of Singapore, a higher place among tropical fruits, than we would give to the far famed mangustin.

Another fruit indigenous to the Straits, and for which most persons, the natives more especially, entertain a remarkable predilection, is the durian. Of this fruit Dr. Ward, in his "Medical Topography of the Straits", observes, "This fruit is well known from the description of travellers; those who have overcome the prejudice excited by the disagreeable foetid odour of the external shell, reckon it delicious. From experience I can pronounce it the most luscious and the most fascinating fruit in the universe . . ."

We made a great effort to eat this fruit a few days ago. There was nothing amiss with it when it was first placed before us, but no sooner had we divided the shell that holds that delicious pulp, whose exquisite flavour, as we are told, no human art could equal, than our olfactory nerves were assailed with such an effluvia, as well nigh scared us from our propriety. We could go no further . . . we are not ashamed to admit that our natural repugnance for offensive smells must ever prevent our acquiring a relish for this popular fruit.

A BENGAL CIVILIAN
Rambles in Java and the Straits in 1852
(1853)

1854

An Eastern Scene

*Lieutenant A.W. Habersham of the U.S. Navy was a member of the
North Pacific Surveying and Exploring Expedition 1853–56, sent out
by the U.S. Government. At the time, Habersham kept a journal
from which he quoted freely in his later published account.*

After we had been working some two months, the schooner was
ordered to proceed to Singapore, (distant some three hundred miles), to
communicate with the consul, and return as soon as possible. I was so
fortunate as to remain by her during the trip, and on the 7th of March
we found ourselves at anchor off that city.

While Stevens and myself were stepping into a sampan to go on shore,
a light row-boat pulled alongside, in the centre of which stood a very
black Hindoo with a very white turban around his head. He introduced
himself as follows:– "Me Mohammed! – consul-man. Plenty, oh! *plenty*
letter at consul-house for American man-war." But I will say nothing
more of letters; for there was but one for me, and that a half-year old.

We went to the consul's, and thence to the London Hotel, where we
tasted a bottle of sour Bordeaux, drank another of pale ale, and engaged
a room at two dollars a day.

I will be brief in regard to our treatment while in that city. I will only
say that, from the governor down to the ship-chandlers, there seemed to
be a determination that we should never dine at the hotel. Such hospitality I never saw before. In company with the consul, we went to call
upon the governor's family shortly after our arrival.

"We got into our undress uniform, then into a carriage, which we
hired for a dollar a day, and after a five minutes' drive commenced
winding around the hill which towers over the city, and upon the crest
of which stands the palace. This spiral road was a mile or more in
length, and wormed through the tastefully laid-out grounds in the centre
of which stood the edifice. We drove through groves of the fragrant nut-

meg and of the luscious mangosteen, crushing the precious fruit under our wheels and breathing the perfumed air that cooled our brows. It fully realized my idea of an Eastern scene: it was one of those drives that flush the cheek of the invalid and diffuse a dreamy languor through the frame of health; it was grand. As we thus wound around the hill, we gazed upon a constantly-changing scene. We saw the whole of Singapore twice over; for the palace rose out of the centre of the town almost, overlooking every thing. Thus we looked down upon the city by piecemeal at first, and finally, upon reaching the summit, took in 'the whole' at a revolving glance, – the city, the bay, the opposite land, the back-country with its dense jungle, and the immediate grounds around our feet. This also was grand.

"We were ushered into the reception-room by a fancifully-liveried native, and were soon after met by the ladies. We found Mrs. and Miss Butterworth most accomplished personages, and passed a pleasant fifteen minutes. They showed us a stone which had lately been brought from a mountain in the island of Banca, (one of those around which we were surveying,) and which exerted a powerful influence over the needle: every one called it a loadstone. Stevens, having found that it would not attract a *cambric*-needle, pronounced it a singular iron-ore; and such subsequently proved to be its nature."

We had been riding around in our one-dollar vehicle to see the sights. Here is one of them, a Chinese temple:–

"As we entered through the massive stone-work, we were followed by a dozen or more loafing Chinamen, who stopped their gambling (gambling in the very porch of their temple!) to watch our movements. We were very respectful at first, for fear of alarming their jealousy, throwing away our cigars and taking off our hats. These loafers, however, motioned us to light other cigars and to resume our covering, and were so attentive as to bring us fire. They also spit on the smooth and polished floor, to show us, I suppose, that we were at liberty to do likewise. In addition to all this, they advanced to the chancel and commenced a series of violent bends and gesticulations for our information. They were showing us how they paid their devotions. They stood before a massive altar, decked out after the manner of the Romish Church, having upon its right a colossal statue of a very benign old gentleman, and upon its left a similar one with the most hideously-diabolical expression that I ever saw. The one on the right shone as the concentration of every thing good, and extended his left hand in an endless blessing. He of the left – the rampant power of evil – settled his gaze of eternal hate

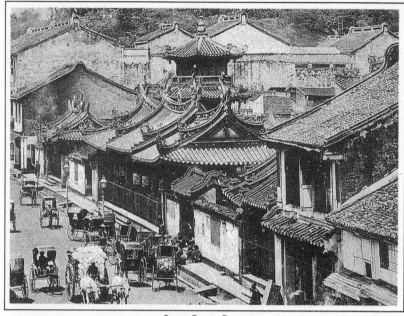

SOUTH BRIDGE ROAD

and defiance upon the averted eye of the first, and grasped a bleeding heart in his uplifted hand. It was to this latter that all the devotions were addressed: no one looked at the other. We gave them a half-crown for putting themselves into a perspiration by their furious pantomime, and continued our drive."

A.W. HABERSHAM
My Last Cruise **(1878)**

58

In the Chinese Bazaar

*Alfred Russel Wallace was a leading English naturalist who, indepen-
dently of Darwin and while in Borneo, devised a theory of evolution
by natural selection. His expedition to the East lasted eight years and
covered 14,000 miles around the region. Some 125,000 specimens
(ranging from mammals to insects) were collected, a good number from
Singapore. Wallace visited Singapore several times, staying with his
friend, a Jesuit missionary.*

By far the most conspicuous of the various kinds of people in
Singapore, and those which most attract the stranger's attention, are the
Chinese, whose numbers and incessant activity give the place very much
the appearance of a town in China. The Chinese merchant is generally
a fat round-faced man with an important and business-like look. He
wears the same style of clothing (loose white smock, and blue or black
trousers) as the meanest coolie, but of finer materials, and is always clean
and neat; and his long tail tipped with red silk hangs down to his heels.
He has a handsome warehouse or shop in town and a good house in the
country. He keeps a fine horse and gig, and every evening may be seen
taking a drive bareheaded to enjoy the cool breeze. He is rich, he owns
several retail shops and trading schooners, he lends money at high
interest and on good security, he makes hard bargains and gets fatter
and richer every year.

In the Chinese bazaar are hundreds of small shops in which a miscel-
laneous collection of hardware and dry goods are to be found, and
where many things are sold wonderfully cheap. You may buy gimlets at
a penny each, white cotton thread at four balls for a halfpenny, and
penknives, corkscrews, gunpowder, writing-paper, and many other
articles as cheap or cheaper than you can purchase them in England.
The shopkeeper is very good-natured; he will show you everything he
has, and does not seem to mind if you buy nothing.. He bates a little,

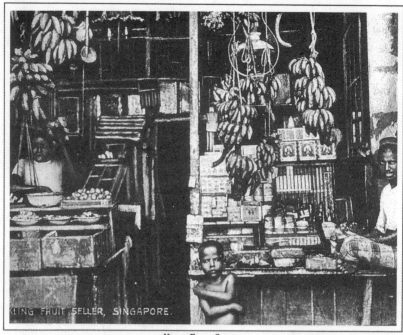

KLING FRUIT SELLER

but not so much as the Klings, who almost always ask twice what they are willing to take. If you buy a few things of him, he will speak to you afterwards every time you pass his shop, asking you to walk in and sit down, or take a cup of tea, and you wonder how he can get a living where so many sell the same trifling articles. The tailors sit *at* a table, not *on* one; and both they and the shoemakers work well and cheaply. The barbers have plenty to do, shaving heads and cleaning ears; for which latter operation they have a great array of little tweezers, picks, and brushes. In the outskirts of the town are scores of carpenters and blacksmiths. The former seem chiefly to make coffins and highly painted and decorated clothes-boxes. The latter are mostly gun-makers, and bore the barrels of guns by hand, out of solid bars of iron. At this tedious operation they may be seen every day, and they manage to finish off a gun with a flint lock very handsomely. All about the streets are sellers of water, vegetables, fruit, soup, and agar-agar (a jelly made of seaweed), who have many cries as unintelligible as those of London. Others carry a portable cooking-apparatus on a pole balanced by a table at the other end, and serve up a meal of shellfish, rice, and vegetables for two or three halfpence; while coolies and boatmen waiting to be hired are everywhere to be met with.

In the interior of the island the Chinese cut down forest trees in the jungle, and saw them up into planks; they cultivate vegetables, which they bring to market; and they grow pepper and gambir, which form important articles of export. The French Jesuits have established missions among these inland Chinese, which seem very successful. I lived for several weeks at a time with the missionary at Bukit-tima, about the centre of the island, where a pretty church has been built and there are about 300 converts. While there, I met a missionary who had just arrived from Tonquin, where he had been living for many years. The Jesuits still do their work thoroughly as of old. In Cochin China, Tonquin, and China, where all Christian teachers are obliged to live in secret, and are liable to persecution, expulsion, and sometimes death, every province, even those farthest in the interior, has a permanent Jesuit mission establishment, constantly kept up by fresh aspirants, who are taught the languages of the countries they are going to at Penang or Singapore. In China there are said to be near a million converts; in Tonquin and Cochin China, more than half a million. One secret of the success of these missions is the rigid economy practised in the expenditure of the funds. A missionary is allowed about 30*l.* a year, on which he lives in whatever country he may be. This renders it possible to support a large number of missionaries with very limited means; and the natives, seeing their teachers living in poverty and with none of the luxuries of life, are convinced that they are sincere in what they teach, and have really given up home and friends and ease and safety for the good of others. No wonder they make converts, for it must be a great blessing to the poor people among whom they labour to have a man among them to whom they can go in any trouble or distress, who will comfort and advise them, who visits them in sickness, who relieves them in want, and who devotes his whole life to their instruction and welfare.

My friend at Bukit-tima was truly a father to his flock. He preached to them in Chinese every Sunday, and had evenings for discussion and conversation on religion during the week. He had a school to teach their children. His house was open to them day and night. If a man came to him and said, "I have no rice for my family to eat to-day," he would give him half of what he had in the house, however little that might be. If another said, "I have no money to pay my debt," he would give him half

61

the contents of his purse, were it his last dollar. So, when he was himself in want, he would send to some of the wealthiest among his flock, and say, "I have no rice in the house," or "I have given away my money, and am in want of such and such articles." The result was that his flock trusted and loved him, for they felt sure that he was their true friend, and had no ulterior designs in living among them.

Insects were exceedingly abundant and very interesting, and every day furnished scores of new and curious forms. In about two months I obtained no less than 700 species of beetles, a large proportion of which were quite new, and among them were 130 distinct kinds of the elegant Longicorns (Cerambycidæ), so much esteemed by collectors. Almost all these were collected in one patch of jungle, not more than a square mile in extent, and in all my subsequent travels in the East I rarely if ever met with so productive a spot. This exceeding productiveness was due in part no doubt to some favourable conditions in the soil, climate, and vegetation, and to the season being very bright and sunny, with suffi-cient showers to keep everything fresh. But it was also in a great measure dependent, I feel sure, on the labours of the Chinese wood-cutters. They had been at work here for several years, and during all that time had furnished a continual supply of dry and dead and decaying leaves and bark, together with abundance of wood and sawdust, for the nourish-ment of insects and their larvæ. This had led to the assemblage of a great variety of species in a limited space, and I was the first naturalist who had come to reap the harvest they had prepared. In the same place, and during my walks in other directions, I obtained a fair collection of butterflies and of other orders of insects, so that on the whole I was quite satisfied with these my first attempts to gain a knowledge of the Natural History of the Malay Archipelago.

ALFRED RUSSEL WALLACE
The Malay Archipelago (1869)

1856-57

Wild Pariah Dogs

These glimpses of Singapore life were written by an English boy in his teens. George Mildmay Dare, son of a sea captain, lived with his family on the corner of Beach Road where the Raffles Hotel now stands. After schooling in England he returned to Singapore and began work in the offices of Syme & Co. (His final reference is to the Indian Mutiny which started in Bengal in February 1857.)

July 1856. – I had a tremendous spill the other day on the Esplanade, when riding home from office, owing to a brute of a pariah dog chasing the pony and getting under his feet and throwing him down. I was thrown, too, and dreadfully shaken and stunned. These pariahs are dreadful nuisances, and the convicts do not half carry out the law on the first three days of every month, which are set aside for killing dogs. . . .

On the Queen's Birthday we went over to Blakan Mati to fish, in a rowing boat. There is very little to shoot on this island; it used to be called in English 'Barren Isle'; but some of the islands are full of pigeon and wild pig, and I hope to go down as soon as I can get another gun, for I have sold the last bought on account of its being German, and likely to burst, as most of them do. . . . By the way, while shooting on the jungly swamps beyond the racecourse and the Hindoo cremation grounds last Friday, I came across the remains of three dead bodies on an open plain amid the swamps, evidently belonging to a class of Hindoos who burn their dead, first covering the corpses with wood, to which they set fire. Two of the bodies were charred to cinders, but on the third the fire had apparently gone out, and there he was, only slightly grilled and smelling horribly. Wild pariah dogs had run away with one of his legs and part of his thigh, of which I found the bones some distance off, partly devoured. I think the police ought to put a stop to such infernal practices! The effect of this nasty sight was sufficient to

63

give the Malay who accompanied me such a shock that he swore that he saw their three ghosts! and there was no more shooting that day.

January 1857. – Our native population are in a very disturbed state, on account of the recently passed Conservancy and Police Acts. Late in the afternoon of the 31st ultimo, it was known to a few that the Chinese had resolved to close their shops, and on that day, it is said, monster meetings of the Chinese secret societies took place in the rural districts.

New Year's Day being a holiday by universal consent, no notice was taken of the shops being closed. On the 2nd they were still all closed, and boatmen, syces, artificers, and coolies all ceased their ordinary occupations – it was a general strike, showing that not only all classes of natives were acting in concert, but that from their doing so simultaneously it must have been a pre-arranged movement. That intimidation was used there is no doubt; the ferry-boatmen were told by some Chinese that if they persisted in ferrying Europeans across the river, the Chinese would put their eyes out at night. Shortly after 6 a.m. the markets were cleared, and by 9 o'clock the streets were crowded with Chinese idlers, who appeared anxious for some opportunity to commence a riot: indeed, just before eight, the Deputy Commissioner of Police and his peons were attacked in Market Street, and repulsed with a few scratches and bruises, and by 10 a.m. all the Europeans had arrived in town and found the strike universal. A public meeting was convened by the Sheriff, the Volunteer Rifle Corps mustered, the troops held in readiness in case of need. The Resident Councillor caused a proclamation to be issued, calling on the people to open their shops, and if they had any cause for complaint, to make it known to the Governor. On Saturday Governor Blundell called the heads of the principal Chinese merchants together, and arranged with them to have a translation made of the Act and circulated amongst the various members of the Chinese community, the former issued being so faulty as to convey quite an erroneous impression of the actual provisions of the law. This had a pacifying effect, and they all opened their shops and pursued their ordinary avocations. Matters are still far from settled; seditious placards in Chinese are still posted about the streets, calling upon the Chinese to rebel against the Europeans and turn them out of the island, and have gone so far as to offer rewards for the heads of the Governor and some of the principal officers of the Court! As may be imagined, no traces of the author of these can be discovered. . . .

February 1857. – Great fears have been lately entertained regarding the convicts, as a Sikh chief Ghurruk Singh, who was a State prisoner some time ago, has been tampering with them, and formed a plan of rising whilst all the Europeans were in church and massacring all. There are from 1,000 to 2,000 convicts of the same class as those now rebels in Bengal, and of which some eighty are Sikhs; so we are all on the look-out for a riot soon. . . .

> **G.M. DARE**
> **Accounts of Singapore Life**
> *One Hundred Years of Singapore* (1921)
> Ed. William Makepeace

1857

Long Tails and Loose Trousers

A journalist and travel writer, Laurence Oliphant had studied law and been called to the Bar. At twenty-eight he accompanied the Earl of Elgin as his Private Secretary on a diplomatic mission to China and Japan. It was while on this mission that Oliphant stopped off in Singapore.

At present there is a population of 70,000 Chinamen in Singapore, and not a single European who understands their language. The consequence is, that, in the absence of any competent interpreter, they are generally ignorant of the designs of Government, and, regarding themselves still as Chinese subjects, are apt to place themselves in an antagonistic attitude whenever laws are passed affecting their peculiar customs. No effort is made to overcome a certain exclusiveness arising hence; and this is fostered by the secret societies, which exercise an important moral influence upon the minds of all, but more particularly the ignorant portion of the population. Were Chinese themselves put into positions of authority under Government, and allowed to share to some extent in the duties and responsibilities of British citizens, which, intellectually speaking, they are quite competent to undertake, – the barrier which now exists between the two races would be partially removed, and the mutual distrust and suspicion engendered by our present system would in all probability quickly disappear. Nor is this mere speculation. We have fortunately in their own empire a perpetual proof before our eyes of that reverence for authority *when judiciously enforced*, which is one of their chief characteristics, and which has for so many centuries been the preservation of its union and one great source of its prosperity.

That the most active, industrious, and enterprising race in the Eastern world should be regarded as a source of weakness, rather than of strength to a community, implies, *primâ facie*, a certain degree of mis-

66

management. The Chinese who have been attracted to Singapore by its freedom from commercial restrictions, and advantages of position, have contributed to make it what it is, the most prosperous settlement in the East; and when we consider their extraordinary acquisitiveness and love of gain, we can hardly suppose that their sympathies with their brethren in China would be sufficiently powerful to induce them wantonly to interrupt a commerce, from which they derive enormous profits, and destroy a mercantile emporium which may be said to be in a great degree their own handiwork, and in which they possess a larger stake than any other class of its community.

To the stranger first arriving in Singapore, nothing can be more striking than the busy aspect which the place presents. Every street swarms with long tails and loose trousers; throughout whole sections of the town are red lintels of the door-posts covered with fantastic characters, which betoken a Chinese owner. At early dawn the incessant hammering, stitching, and cobblering commences, which lasts until nearly midnight; when huge paper lanterns, covered with strange devices, throw a subdued light over rows of half-naked yellow figures, all eagerly engaged in the legitimate process of acquiring dollars by the sweat of their brow. It is impossible to over-estimate the value of such a race, or to rate too highly the importance of placing them in such relations with the governing powers, by the cultivation of a more familiar intercourse, and a certain deference to their habits and prejudices, as should render them contented and trustworthy, as well as profitable, members of society.

LAURENCE OLIPHANT
Narrative of the Earl of Elgin's
Mission to China and Japan (1859)

1860

A Party of Convicts

Colonel Orfeur Cavenagh was the last Governor of the Straits Settlements to be appointed from India. Writing his memoirs in later years he recalled incidents from his days in Singapore.

At all the stations in the Straits there were large convict establishments, at which the system subsequently introduced into Ireland had been enforced for years. Every convict on his arrival was placed in the lowest grade and worked as an ordinary labourer, in irons, for a specified term of years; at the expiration of that period, in the event of his having a sufficiently clear defaulter's-sheet – for every offence, however slight, was duly recorded – he was promoted to a higher class, his fetters were lightened, and if he showed an aptitude for learning any handicraft he was transferred to the workshops and taught some trade. When the second term elapsed, he was in like manner again promoted, and employed as an artificer, receiving, according to his merits, some slight remuneration for his services. At the end of the third period he was raised to the position of a petty officer, and was permitted to leave the precincts of the jail for a short time after working hours. The full term of probation having expired, he was granted a ticket-of-leave, on condition, however, of providing a suitable security, who became bound for his good behaviour. . . .

A very great number of public buildings, amongst them a handsome church at Singapore, were erected entirely by convict labour, whilst by the same means most of the roads throughout the three stations were constructed and kept in order. As a rule the convicts were very well behaved, and shortly after my arrival at Singapore, I was much struck by a remark made by the commissioner of police, who was referring to the case of a lady who had wandered into the jungle and lost her way; and stated that although her husband was much alarmed, as she wore some valuable jewels, the moment he heard that she had fallen in with a

68

party of convicts employed in road-making, he ceased to have any fears for her safety.

The loss of life at Singapore, owing to the destruction caused by tigers, who struck down the Chinese employed in the Gambier and pepper plantations, was at one time very great, the number of persons thus annually destroyed having been estimated by the Commissioner of Police at two hundred. Discussing this subject one day with the Superintendent of Convicts, he mentioned that amongst the prisoners under his charge there were several good shots, and suggested that their services might be utilized towards remedying the evil. Ultimately it was arranged that two parties, of eight men each, should be furnished with arms and ammunition, and sent out into the jungles, where they would be allowed to remain, merely coming in to attend the monthly muster, so long as they succeeded in destroying a tiger every three months, they being at the same time allowed to receive the Government reward as a stimulus to their exertions. The number of tigers soon diminished, and the necessity for the second party ceased. When I left the Straits cases of death from tigers were of rare occurrence. . . .

On the morning of the 10th of May, I went on board two junks, which under an Act for the Suppression of Piracy, had been seized by the police on suspicion of having been engaged in piratical courses. There could be little doubt as to the nature of their calling, for they were heavily armed and well supplied with ammunition, as well as with stinkpots and large jars full of broken glass to be flung from the masthead upon the deck of any vessel attacked so as to drive the crew below. With the prisoners there was a Chinese dog which was let loose upon the police when they boarded, and with the aid of a pig, which drove off the Mahommedans of the party, for a short time completely cleared the deck. . . .

Although on this occasion the junks were released, the suspicions of the police as to their real character proved to be well founded, for shortly after one of them was recognized by a Chinese trader as being the junk that had bèen taken from him by pirates on the coast of China. Although the charge of piracy he brought against one of the crew was dismissed by the magistrates on the ground of want of jurisdiction, the vessel was ordered by the higher court to be restored to its proper owner.

GENERAL SIR ORFEUR CAVENAGH
Reminiscences of an Indian Official (1884)

1864

Amok

*Believing public opinion in England to be largely uninformed about
conditions in the Straits Settlements, John Cameron wrote a detailed
descriptive book to provide the necessary background. He had set up
business in Singapore a few years earlier, and was at the same time
editor of the* Straits Times *newspaper.*

The Chinese barbers' shops are numerous throughout the town: and,
singularly enough, they are marked by variegated poles very much
resembling those used by the same trade at home, only that they are
square and not round. They are generally entirely open to the street,
and the operations are gone through in the most public manner possible. Hair-cutting is never part of these operations, for all the hair that
Chinamen allow to grow on their heads is gathered up into a tail
behind, which is never cut, its length and luxuriance being its chief rec-
ommendation. The tail, however, is opened out, combed, and replaited,
and the head all around, as well as the face, is shaved. While this is
being done, the customers sit poised upon stools, in view of all passers-
by, gazing forward with the same blank stolidity that pervades the faces
of those under operation in any barber's shop at home.

There is probably no city in the world with such a motley crowd of
itinerant vendors of wares, fruits, cakes, vegetables, &c. There are
Malays, generally with fruit; Chinamen with a mixture of all sorts, and
Klings with cakes and different kinds of nuts. Malays and Chinamen
always use the shoulder-stick, having equally-balanced loads suspended
at either end; the Klings, on the contrary, carry their wares on the head
on trays. The travelling cookshops of the Chinese are probably the most
extraordinary of the things that are carried about in this way. They are
suspended on one of the common shoulder-sticks, and consist of a box
on one side and a basket on the other; the former containing a fire and
small copper cauldron for soup; the latter loaded with rice, vermicelli,

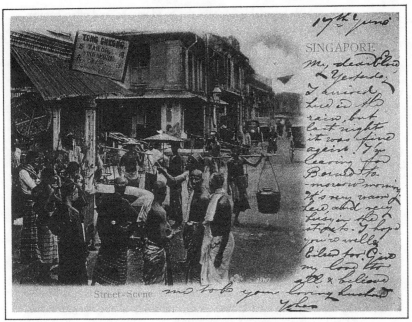

Street-Scene

STREET SCENE

cakes, jellies, and condiments; and though I have never tasted any of their dishes, I have been assured that those they serve up at a moment's notice are most savoury, and that their sweets are delicious. Three cents will purchase a substantial meal of three or four dishes from these itinerant restaurateurs.

Another remarkable feature of the streets, and one which carries the mind away back to a very early period in the history of our own country, is made up of the letter-writers or penny-a-liners, who take up their stalls at various parts of the town. They are always to be seen in the mornings seated composedly at their desks in the verandahs or out in the streets. On their desks or tables are piled several quires of Chinese straw paper, and a small porcelain tablet contains their ink and writing-brushes; pens of any kind are unknown to them. A large – perhaps the largest – section of the Chinese population cannot write for themselves, but all are equally endowed with this amiable feature, that they never forget or neglect the friends they have left behind them in China; and these letter-writers do a large business in making out for the illiterate section epistles which invariably contain the good wishes, and often convey the substantial money gifts, of those who dictate them. When not engaged in taking down the thoughts of others, these penmen generally employ themselves in copying out stock pamphlets, or, it may be, composing original prose or verse suited to the popular taste. But their productions cannot be very deep, for they seem to write away with great facility, even when not copying; and I have never witnessed them in anything like what we term the agonies of composition. As a rule, they are not more intellectual in appearance than their neighbours, though I have remarked one or two who clearly bore the print of letters on their features. The feast times are the busiest seasons with them, when they make out large placards on red paper to adorn the door-posts and lintels of their customers.

In driving through the narrow streets of Singapore, it is at times difficult to avoid running over some of the crowd. The danger of such an accident is increased by the circumstance that Chinamen are ordinarily very deaf – owing, it is believed, to their so frequently having their ears cleaned out by rough steel instruments – and are also very indifferent. If you nearly run over a Chinaman, and he escapes but by a hair's-breadth, the only way he indicates an appreciation of the danger he has escaped is by turning round to you with a good-natured, well-pleased grin on his face. Some of them will even pass on without raising their heads, as if no danger had been incurred. I shall not soon forget one occasion on which I had the misfortune to run over a Chinaman. It was in a four-wheeled Yankee buggy; the horse had taken fright and started off into a canter, and on turning a corner came right up against a Chinaman who was leisurely walking in the centre of the road. The shaft caught him about the shoulder and down he went; all I felt being the bump, bump of the two pair of wheels passing over his body. In a few moments the horse was pulled up, and on approaching the man I saw him still on the ground, but apparently busily engaged about something. When I got up to him I found that the wheels had passed over his waist, cutting his belt in two, attached to which had been a purse containing a handful of copper cents, which were now scattered on the ground, and the man was quietly gathering them up, never having risen since he was run over. He had two long skin wounds across his waist, but they appeared to give him no anxiety whatever compared with the safety of his money.

Like other countries inhabited by Malays and Bugis, Singapore is subjected occasionally to the dangerous practice of amok running. In apparent obedience to some sudden impulse, a Malay, or Bugis, will arm himself with two large *krises*, or daggers, one in each hand, and rushing from his house along generally the most crowded street in the neighbourhood stab at random all who come in his way. As many as fifteen persons have been killed or seriously wounded, and many others slightly hurt by one of these amok runners before he was slain, but the killed always bear a small proportion to the wounded as the strokes of the infatuated man fall promiscuously and are ill-directed. As soon as an amok runner makes his appearance, a warning cry is raised and carried on in advance of him all along the street. On hearing this cry a general rush into the houses is made of all the women and children and of all the men who are not armed – no attempt is made to capture the maniac alive, but he becomes a mark for the musket, spear, or *kris*, of every man who can obtain a favourable opportunity for attack. He ceases to be viewed as human and is hunted down like a wild beast, yet it is surprising how long he will escape the death which is aimed at him from every side. Some of these unfortunate wretches have run the gauntlet of nearly a mile of street that was up in arms against them, and have temporarily evaded destruction, some for hours, and others for days. But the end is inevitable, they refuse to be captured, and are ultimately shot down or stabbed. . . .

It is impossible to give any explanation of the motives which lead to these fatal frenzies. Some have written that they most generally arise from the dejection succeeding an over-indulgence in opium. But the Malays are seldom addicted to the use of that drug, and nearly all the amoks that have occurred in Singapore were run by men who had never tasted it. It seems to me that they are those who from some cause have become disgusted or tired of life and are determined to die, but that as their religion and superstitions prohibit suicide they resolve to provoke death at the hands of others. This may not account for the efforts they apparently make to escape when they have once started, but I would put these efforts down as unpremeditated, and as an obedience to an after-felt yet irresistible instinct of self-preservation. Not many years ago an amok, in which several lives were lost, was run in Campong Java by a Bugis who was known to be a peaceable, well-to-do, industrious man. He was also a very devout Mohammedan, and for nearly twenty-four hours before he started on the amok was intently perusing the Koran. He was not killed, but was stunned by a blow from behind and taken prisoner. He was condemned to be hanged, and suffered death with the greatest indifference. When asked a few minutes before his execution regarding his motive, he said that he had felt his time was come, and that he was irresistibly impelled to seek death in the manner which he did.

To give a correct idea of the everyday life of the European it is necessary rather to distinguish between the unmarried and the married, than between the man of narrow and the man of extended means. Most of the bungalows . . . are about two miles from town; nearly all, at least, are within hearing range of the 68-pounder gun on Fort Canning, the discharge of which each morning at five o'clock ushers in the day. This is the accepted signal of all old residents to start from bed, the younger however, usually indulge in an extra half-hour's slumber. Still, six o'clock generally sees all dressed and out of doors, to enjoy a couple of miles walk or ride through the lovely country roads, in the delicious coolness of morning, before the sun's rays become disagreeably powerful. . . .

On coming home from these morning rounds, the custom is to get into loose, free and easy attire, generally baju and pajamas. A cup of coffee or tea, with biscuit or bread-and-butter and fruit, is then consumed, and the next two hours spent in reading, writing, or lolling about in the verandahs which front each apartment of a house. . . .

At half-past eight the breakfast dressing gong or bell is sounded. A gentleman's toilette in this part of the east is not an elaborate one, and half an hour is ample time for its completion. The bath is its chief feature. Attached to the dressing-room of each bedroom in almost all houses is a bath-room, with brick-tiled floor, containing a large bathing jar holding about sixty or seventy gallons of water. The orthodox manner of bathing is to stand on a small wooden grating close to the jar, and with a hand bucket to dash the water over the body. This is by no means such an unsatisfactory method as to the uninitiated it may appear. The successive shocks to the system which are obtained by the discharge of each bucketful of water, seems to have a much more bracing effect than that of one sudden and continued immersion. Every gentleman has his native boy or body servant, whose sole duty it is to attend upon him personally. While bathing, these boys lay out their master's apparel for the day; so that on coming from the bath a gentleman has little trouble to get himself attired. As to shaving the process is generally performed by itinerant Hindoo barbers, who for the small charge of a dollar or a dollar and a half per month come every morning round to the residences of their customers. The charge is so small, and the saving in trouble so great, that almost all avail themselves of the convenience.

The universal breakfast hour is nine o'clock, and when the bell then rings the whole household assemble, and should there be ladies of the number this is the first time of their appearance. Singapore breakfasts, though tolerably substantial and provided with a goodly array of dishes, are rarely dwelt over long, half an hour, being about the time devoted to them. A little fish, some curry and rice, and perhaps a couple of eggs, washed down with a tumbler or so of good claret, does not take long to get through and yet forms a very fair foundation on which to begin the labours of the day. After breakfast the conveyances drive round to the porch or portico and having received their owners hasten in to town. No matter how many may reside together, each bachelor has generally his own "turn-out;" and for half an hour every morning the two bridges leading across the river into town present an endless string of these rather motley vehicles – by no means an uninteresting spectacle. . . .

Arrived in town, ten minutes or a quarter of an hour are usually spent in going the rounds of the square to learn the news of the morning. . . . As scarcely a day passes without the arrival of a steamer with news from England, China, India, or from some interesting point in the neighbour-hood, there is always ample material for an animated exchange of ideas and information on leading topics, whether they be European politics, the war in America, the position of affairs in China, the combined action at Japan, the affairs of India, Java, Borneo, the administration of the local Government, or the condition and prospects of the adjacent markets.

This sort of congress takes place between the first arrival in town and ten or half-past ten o'clock. At that hour business has commenced and continues in full force till tiffin time, or one o'clock; and certainly it is gone through in quite as smart and active a manner as at home. The climate, though it may produce a greater languor in the evening, has apparently no such effect during the day. There is not much out-of-door bustle; but still when occasion requires the folks post about the square under the midday sun at a lively pace and with apparent impunity.

Tiffin time does not bring the luxurious abandonment to the table which it does in Java; people in Singapore are more moderate in their indulgence, yet some show of a meal is in most cases made; a plate of curry and rice and some fruit or it may be a simple biscuit with a glass of beer or claret. Half an hour's relaxation too is generally indulged in, and as the daily newspaper comes out about this hour, there is a goodly

75

flocking either to the exchange or the public godowns in the square for a perusal of it. . . .

Business hours are not particularly severe, and by half-past four or five o'clock most of the mercantile houses have got through their work. But only a few proceed direct home at this hour; the greater number, at least of the younger members of the community, resort to the fives-court or the cricket-ground on the esplanade. . . . The game is well-known at home, and I need not describe it further than to say that it is a kind of rackets, but that the hands instead of bats are used to play up the ball and that consequently the exercise is much more severe. It is really surprising, in a temperature seldom ranging at the hour the game is played below 82°, to see those who have gone through a fair day's work at the desk come here and doff their vests, coats, and shirts to an hour or an hour and a half of about the most severe exercise in which it is possible to engage; and this too in an unroofed building with the rays of the sun if not directly beating down, at least reflected in fierce glare from the whitewashed walls. And yet medical men attribute the extreme good health of the residents to this continued exercise indulged in, begun by the morning walk at sunrise and ending with cricket or fives at sunset. Cricket is of course precisely the same game in Singapore as it is at home.

But there are two evenings in the week when the whole European community may generally be seen upon the esplanade, whether or not they be fives or cricket-players, and these are band evenings, generally Tuesdays and Fridays. The band, which is that of the regiment on the station at the time, or from one of the men-of-war which occasionally visit the port, plays on a raised mound on the centre of the esplanade green. The chains which protect the green on ordinary occasions are on these evenings let down, and carriages, horsemen, and pedestrians are alike admitted to the greensward. Gathered round the band in a tolerably broad circle are the beauty and fashion of the place. The ladies, to whom almost all the other outdoor amusements are denied, partake at least in this, and though the ruddy glow of the colder latitudes has fled from most cheeks, still there supervenes a languid softness which is more interesting and perhaps more beautiful. The pretty pale-faced European children too may on these occasions be seen tripping about in playfulness a little less boisterous, but quite as cheerful as is witnessed at home. The band plays from half-past five till half-past six, at which hour it is all but dark, when the carriages make for home in a long string, gradually falling off one by one as the various residences are reached.

Except on band nights however, most of the commercial and all of the official world retire home a little before six o'clock. Arrived there, probably a glass of sherry and bitters will anticipate the refreshing process of dressing for dinner. . . .

Dinner in Singapore is not the light airy meal which might reasonably be imagined from the nature of the climate; on the contrary, it is quite as substantial a matter of fact as in the very coldest latitudes. The difference is not that the substantials are fewer, but that the luxuries are more numerous. Indeed the every-day dinner of Singapore, were it not for the waving punkahs, the white jackets of the gentlemen, and the gauzy dresses of the ladies, the motley array of native servants, each standing behind his master's or mistress's chair, and the goodly display of argand lamps, might not unreasonably be mistaken for some more special occasion at home. Soup and fish generally both precede the substantials, which are of a solid nature, consisting of roast beef or mutton, turkey or capon, supplemented by side-dishes of tongue, fowl, cutlets, or such like, together with an abundant supply of vegetables, including potatoes nearly equal to English ones grown in China or India, and also cabbages from Java. The substantials are invariably followed by curry and rice which forms a characteristic feature of the tables of Singapore, and though Madras and Calcutta have been long famed for the quality of their curries, I nevertheless think that those of the Straits exceed any of them in excellence. There are usually two or more different kinds placed on the table, and accompanying them are all manner of sambals or native pickles and spices, which add materially to the piquancy of the dish.

During the progress of the substantials and of the curry and rice, the usual beverage is beer, accompanied by a glass or two of pale sherry. . . .

To curry and rice succeeds generally some sort of pudding or preserve, but sweets have not the same temptation here as at home. Very good cheese however is obtained in fortnightly supplies by the overland steamers, and, as good fresh butter is always to be had, this part of dinner is well enjoyed, accompanied as it is by no illiberal allowance of excellent pale ale. But it is in the luxuriance of the dessert perhaps more than anything else that the tables of Singapore are to be distinguished, and it is little wonder that it should be so; for there is no season of the year at which an abundance of fruit cannot be obtained. Pineapple may be considered the stock fruit of the island, and one or two splendid specimens of these generally adorn the table.

There are plantains, ducoos, mangoes, rambutans, pomeloes, and mangosteens; the latter fruit is peculiar to the Straits of Malacca and to Java, and so great is its fame that to India or China no present or gift from Singapore is more acceptable than a basket of them. . . . But though dessert generally makes a finer display than any other part of dinner, it is not that to which most attention is directed. A cigar and a glass or two of sherry after the ladies are gone, and dinner is over.

Many of the residences have billiard-rooms attached, in which case the usual custom is to retire there after dinner. Where no billiard-room is within reach, a chat in the verandah, a little meditation, or perhaps a book passes the hours pleasantly enough until bedtime. And as dinner is seldom over before eight o'clock, and the usual hour for rest is ten, it is not a very long interval between them that has to be disposed of.

JOHN CAMERON
Our Tropical Possessions in Malayan India (1865)

A Chinese Burglar

John Thomson was a Fellow of the Royal Geographical Society which had been founded in 1830 to advance geographical knowledge through exploration and research. He was in the Straits Settlements between the years 1861 and 1865, residing for a period in Singapore.

If we knew nothing of Chinese clanship and Chinese guilds, we should think it strange that the wealthier Chinamen are rarely made the victims of the great gang robberies that, during my time, used frequently to occur. These robberies are perpetrated by bands of ruffians numbering at times as many as a hundred strong, who surround and pillage a house that is always the residence of a foreigner. Chinese thieves are thorough experts at their profession, adopting the most ingenious devices to attain their infamous ends. I recollect a burglary which once took place at a friend's house, when the thief found his way into the principal bedroom, and deliberately used up half a box of matches before he could get the candle to light. His patience being rewarded at last, he proceeded with equal coolness in the plunder of the apartment, not forgetting to search beneath the pillow, where he secured a revolver and watch. These Chinese robbers are reported to be able to stupify their victims by using some narcotic known only to themselves. . . .

The Malays have told me of cases where, as they averred, the cunning Chinese thief passes the doorway of the house to be pillaged, and tosses in a handful of rice impregnated with some aromatic drug. This drug soon sends the inmates off into a deep repose, from which they will seldom awaken till long after the robber has finished his undertaking, and that in the complete and deliberate style which suits the taste of the Chinese.

. . . When they have a daring burglary on hand, they go quite naked, with the body oiled all over, and the queue coiled up into a knob at the back of the head, and stuck full of needles on every side. The following

79

adventure with a Chinese burglar befell a friend of mine. About mid-night, as he lay awake in his bed, with the lamp extinguished and the windows opened to admit the air, he saw a dark figure clamber over his window-sill and enter the apartment. He kept himself motionless, till the thief, believing all to be safe, had stolen into the centre of the room, and then sprang out of bed and seized the intruder. Both were powerful men, and a furious struggle consequently ensued; but the robber had the advantage, for his only covering was a coat of oil; so that at last, slipping like an eel from the grasp of his antagonist, he made a plunge at the window, and was about to drop into the garden beneath when his pursuer, with a final effort, managed to catch him by the tail. The tail, stuck full of needles, and alas! a false one too, came away by the weight of the fall, and was left a worthless trophy in the hands of the European whom its proprietor had vainly tried to rob.

The Singapore residents have devised many amusements for them-selves. They have their clubs, their bowling-alleys and fives' courts, and their race course. Picnics are numerous, and the frequent gatherings at private houses are pleasantly diversified by performances at the Theatre, and concerts in the Town Hall.

There used also to be a sporting Club, and more than once I have been out tiger-hunting with its members, but I never encountered any-thing more formidable than a deer....

I once went out pig-shooting with a party, to spend the night in the jungle. We put up in a small watch-house, one of many such which are elevated in the jungle, standing on posts of bamboo about ten feet above the ground, and with a platform or flooring not more than six feet square; above is a thatched roof of palm-leaves. We were a party of four, one of us an American gentleman, the finest shot in the Straits – or supposed to be, by many. Having proceeded to a clearing close to the jungle, we entered on the business of laying in wait – a ceremony by no means the most enjoyable among those incident to the sport. These wild pigs feed in herds by night; so we spread a store of pine-apples on the ground, and then, with such patience as we could muster, we tarried to see what fortune would send us. Our clothes were of the thinnest; the stinging ants never tired of their attacks; while the bloodthirsty mos-quitos buzzing about our heads, and diving into our ears, supported the invading armies of ants by light incursions, which harried our necks and heads, so that it became most difficult to maintain the silence essential to the success of our expedition. At length, after three protracted hours of weary watching and unreproachful agony, we heard the distant snorts and grunts that heralded the approach of the swine. As turtle to aldermen, so are dainty pine-apples to these denizens of the jungle. They had got scent of our bait, and were moving in our direction. They came on, but not incautiously. Now they come on in bristling phalanx, and snort for the encounter, and now they grunt a signal to halt. Swift and agile I already knew them to be; but now, too, I discovered in them such a happy combination of boldness and prudence that I thought if undomesticated pigs could but over come their greediness, they might rank among the noblest creatures of the forest. But, alas! in this case as in too many unhappy instances of the past, the prospect of a rich feast was a temptation too great for their grovelling nature! On they came crashing towards us, through the jungle in front. We grasped our rifles so as to sweep the clearing, and awaited the charge of the foe; but unhappily preferring American to English institutions, they swept suddenly round to the field commanded by the doughty sportsman from the United States.

Then a rifle report, a yelling and a grunting, followed by the hasty pattering of the feet of our enemies, as they turned their trotters in full flight; and lo! when we hurried to the spot, expecting to find at least one victim to the trusty weapon of our friend, we, to our dismay, discovered him seated on the ground nursing one leg, and threatening in most unparliamentary language Baboo his native servant, who laughed, and lurked behind a tree. It appeared that the leader of the herd, a huge hog, had charged our friend before he could take aim, had run through between his legs and toppled him over in the act of firing, and carried his followers into the jungle unscathed. Disappointed, but not discouraged, we determined to keep watch, in the hope that the pigs would return. So we fixed Baboo as a sentinel on the bamboo ladder of the hut, in such a way that he would fall off if he went to sleep, and then ourselves retired to rest. When we awoke the hot sun was shining brightly. Baboo, coiled round the ladder like a snake, was still fast asleep, and the pigs, undisturbed, had feasted upon the pine-apples beneath our feet.

J. THOMSON
*The Straits of Malacca, Indo-China
and China or Ten Years' Travels,
Adventures and Residence Abroad*
(1875)

1869

A Scene of Terror

E.D.G. *Prime came from New York and was travelling around the world "mainly for the recovery of health". Here he describes the voyage from Hong Kong to Singapore during the monsoon - not quite, as it turns out, what the doctor ordered.*

Before embarking . . . we were assured that at this season of the year, the last of November, we should have a delightful passage to Singapore, with only enough of the northeast monsoon to keep the air from stagnating, and the sea from becoming like molten glass. But I have learned to put little faith in predictions of the weather, even by sailors, having been obliged so often to interpret prophecies by contraries. . . .

Among the passengers we numbered eight Americans, who took possession of one side of the deck, which, in anticipation of hot weather, was to be our home day and night for nearly a fortnight. On the opposite side of the deck were several wealthy Jews, the ladies in a blaze of diamonds as they came on deck; three Parsees, two of whom, a gentleman and his wife, were our fellow-passengers on crossing the Pacific Ocean. Two Armenians subsequently came on board. The deck-passengers were Chinese, Bengalese, Hindoos, Mohammedans, and I do not know what all. We did not want for variety; but, strange to say, notwithstanding the numerous nationalities, and the fact that the most of our passengers were residents of Oriental countries, the only language that was ordinarily spoken was English. . . .

We had but fairly got out of the harbor and from under the shelter of the headlands when we caught the monsoon, blowing fresh and strong. It upset all our calculations in more senses than one, but the sweet assurance was given us that the wind would go down as we got farther south. On the contrary, the farther south we ran the more heavily the wind blew. There was one consolation - it was a fair wind, but as it increased, the huge waves came chasing us from behind, threatening all the while to overwhelm us. Not being able to move about much of the time, we sat or lay on deck watching the great seas as they towered above the stern, coming on with all their force, as if determined the next time to pounce upon us and wash us all from the deck; but our ship never failed to obey the law of gravitation which gives the highest place to the lighter body, and just at the critical moment she would lift her stern gracefully and allow the swell to pass underneath. This she continued to do for five days, the monsoon increasing all the while, and tossing us up and down most inconveniently.

In the evening of the fifth day out, when we were within about two degrees of the equator, dark clouds were seen gathering in the west, which soon overspread the sky and the sea, the blackness of which was relieved only by fierce flashes of lightning. Presently the rain came down in a tropical deluge; and while the elements were all in wild commotion, the engine suddenly stopped, the ship swung round into the trough of the sea as helpless as a log, and then commenced that awful rolling of the vessel which is far more terrible than driving before or even facing a storm. The heat was too great for us to go below, and we preferred to remain on deck, sheltered only by an awning, and take the chances of the storm; but as the ship rolled heavily from one side to the other, as if about to roll completely over, we were thrown about or compelled to cling fast to whatever was within reach. Some of the passengers were overcome with terror, expecting by the next lurch of the ship to be pitched into the sea. One poor Jewess, who came on board with a fortune on her person in the shape of diamonds and emeralds, shrieked aloud and called upon God to save her. It was to all of us more or less a scene of terror, aggravated by the absolute blackness of darkness that surrounded us. . . .

The moment that the engine stopped I comprehended the cause. I had learned from the captain that we were drawing near a rocky part of the China Sea, in which were several islands, and in the thick darkness and descending torrents of rain it was impossible to see the course; we might at any moment strike a rock or run ashore; it was safer to let the ship drift than to drive her with the engine. The storm of rain became so severe that we were at length compelled to go below, but all night long the ship was starting and stopping, and when the morning came, instead of being to the west of Bintang Island, as we should have been, we had drifted with the currents thirty miles to the east. The morning light was

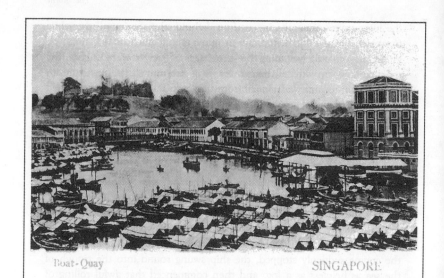

Boat-Quay   SINGAPORE

BOAT QUAY

very pleasant to the eyes, and so was the sight of Singapore, with its beautiful groves of palm, and its substantial buildings stretching along the shore for one or two miles.

E.D.G. PRIME
Around the World: Sketches of Travel (1874)

84

1869

The Chinaman's Garden

Charles Coffin and his wife, Americans on a world tour, visited the famous Whampoa Gardens in Singapore. The Whampoa fortune had been made through supplying stores to British naval vessels calling at the harbour, and for many years the Gardens were a major local attraction.

"Don't fail to see the Chinaman's garden," is the injunction of a gentleman on the steamer. Taking a carriage, we ride through the town, past the government buildings, – large and imposing edifices, looming grandly from the bay, – past two very pretty churches, and residences of merchants, surrounded by well kept grounds, shaded with tropical trees, and beautified by gorgeous flowers of every hue. Upon the road we meet crowds of Chinese, going to or returning from market; some halting at the tea-shops to drink their favorite beverage, or at the opium saloons to whiff the fumes of the stupefying drug.

Never rode we through an avenue so beautiful as that leading to the "Whampoa Gardens." Stately palms, wild almonds, tall, feathery bamboos, and trees of unknown name, line the roadway, spreading out their branches overhead, their trunks wreathed with creeping plants. Orchids and wild heliotrope bloom in the thick hedges: shrubs, plants, vines, in endless variety, broad and narrow leaved, ovate, heart-shaped, trifoliate, – leaf and flowers filling the air with odors new and strange, and almost overpowering.

A ride of about two miles brings us to the residence of a Chinaman who has made a large fortune by trade at Singapore, and who, instead of returning to his native land, as most of his countrymen are in the habit of doing, has made this his permanent home. He loves floriculture, and has spent a great deal of money in fitting up his residence and the grounds around it. A tall fellow, with thin face, lantern-jaws, long pigtail, wearing a blue cotton tunic and flowing trousers and Chinese hat,

85

escorts us through the grounds, to which we have free admission. The proprietor is sick, otherwise he would himself show us the rare tropical plants and flowers.

The grounds are not laid out in accordance with the rules of landscape gardening given by English and American florists. The premises contain a dozen acres, – gardens within gardens, – with arbors, tea-houses, and canals, and tanks stocked with goldfish. There are straight paths, winding walks, and labyrinths, a wonderful variety of tropical vegetation, – a place where the florist or botanist might find unspeakable pleasure. Our conductor brings us to a section of the grounds where dogs, dragons, hobgoblins, and crocodiles, with great goggle eyes, stare at us, – fashioned from a twining shrub, that is hedged in and clipped off, trained on wires, and thus tortured into fantastic shapes.

Passing through one of the tea-houses, we find that the proprietor has Italian vases, French clocks, Japanese carved work, windows of German stained glass, floors of English encaustic tiles, flower-pots from the potteries of his native land, arranged with little taste or order. A Chinaman's ideas of the artistic are grotesque. The pictures which we see on China-ware are excellent representations of Chinese art. They have not advanced beyond the child's plain surface drawing, and have no comprehension of the rules of perspective.

The chief attractions of the garden are the monster *Victoria regias*, which here reach their full development in the open air. Flocks of water-fowl are sitting on the leaves of the plants, which are large and strong enough to bear up a child.

Here we behold the gigantic fan-palm, flourishing with wonderful vigor, the stems of the leaves radiating from the tall trunk like the sticks of a fan, each leaf seven or eight feet in length. . . .

On one side of the garden is a hospital for hogs. The owner of the grounds is a believer in the Buddhist religion, and holds to the transmigration of souls. Entering the pigsty, we behold about a dozen fat porkers. The owner keeps them in excellent condition; they have enough to eat and are well cared for, inasmuch as the spirit of his father may be inhabiting one of them, his grandfather another!

CHARLES CARLETON COFFIN
Our New Way Round The World (1869)

Into the Interior

To study "Man and Nature in the various lands of southern and eastern Asia" – this was Frank Vincent's purpose in travelling. Altogether he spent some three years in the region. (The telegraph to Hong Kong, mentioned here, was opened a few months after Vincent's visit.)

Like Malacca, very little of the town or city of Singapore appears from the sea . . . We steam past two or three war vessels, two telegraph steamers (which are only awaiting orders from London to commence laying a wire from here to Hong Kong), and by some thirty or forty merchant ships of all nations to our anchorage in the crescent-shaped roadstead about a mile from the town. We engage a Malay *prow* to take us ashore, and are landed near the *Hotel d'Europe*, to which our good captain has recommended us. This hotel we find to be very large and comfortable, situated in the midst of beautiful gardens, facing "the green," and commanding a fine view of the straits, the large island of Bintang in the distance, and the Chinese junks and foreign shipping in the harbour. Attached to the establishment, which is kept by a German, is that "peculiar institution" an American bar-room, where California mixed drinks are served, and there is besides a "regular down east Boston Arctic soda-water fountain;" a billiard-room; and a reading-room, where one will find papers and journals, in four or five languages, from New York, London, Bombay, Calcutta, Batavia, Hong Kong, Shanghae, Yokohama, and San Francisco. . . .

One day we visited Fort Canning to obtain a general view of Singapore. This fort, built upon a small pyramid-shaped hill, about 200 feet in height, and just back of the town, mounts, among numerous guns of smaller calibre, some few 68-pounders, and is garrisoned by 300 British and 700 Sepoy troops. Singapore is divided into a Malay, Chinese, and European "town," or quarter; it is too irregular to present a handsome

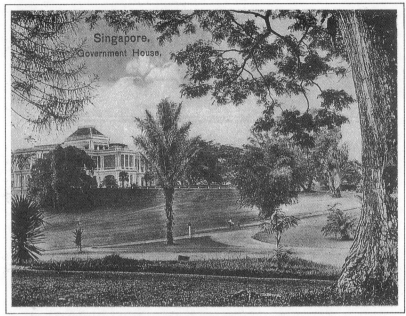

GOVERNMENT HOUSE

appearance, but the view of the shipping in the harbour and the distant islands is rather impressive. . . . The Governor's house is a large brick and stucco building on the summit of a little knoll, perhaps half a mile inland from Fort Canning. Were it not for its immense cupola it would be mistaken for a Government department or office of some kind, and, as it is, the second storey, composed entirely of arches and Venetian blinds, and the upper storey formed of pillars and Venetians, present a very ugly appearance. There are few trees about the house, so that it receives the entire force of both sun and rain, and, excepting only when a strong breeze is blowing, it must be a very uncomfortable residence. . . .

We drove several times, while in Singapore, into the interior of the island, *via* Orchard Road and River Valley Road, on which are situated the European bungalows, or country houses, from two to four miles from town. Orchard Road seems to be the most popular as a residence. After leaving town it passes through a narrow valley, with a series of little hillocks on either hand, and upon which many houses have been built. The road is very pretty, being lined by tall bamboo hedges and trees which, uniting above, form a complete shade . . . Beyond the residences are the remains of many nutmeg plantations (the nutmeg for some reason or other will not flourish in Singapore), then succeeds a strip of thin jungle, then the Chinese pepper and gambier plantations, and then comes the jungle in earnest, with its gigantic trees, creepers, orchids, parasites, and fallen or decayed trees, plants, and vegetables. . . .

Cocoa-nut oil is a large item of export from Singapore. Dr. Little, an English gentleman and an old resident, to whom I was so fortunate as to bring letters of introduction, called one morning at the hotel to take me in his buggy to a large cocoa-nut plantation, owned partly by himself and five miles distant from the town. The estate is nearly a mile square, embracing about six hundred acres, situated near the sea shore, and the soil, at least as far as the roots penetrate, is entirely composed of sand. The trees are planted in rows each way about twenty feet apart, and are of all ages and sizes. Cocoa-nuts are raised principally for their oil, though rope is made from the husks, and some quantity of them is exported for food. We walked for some time beneath the trees, and then, re-entering the buggy, drove to a distant part of the plantation where there was a coir-rope manufactory. The European manager was kind enough to explain the different processes of manufacture, which are extremely simple. . . . Nearly 200 Malays and Chinese were employed in this establishment, which "turns out" about 25,000 pounds of rope per annum. This kind of rope, though extensively used by vessels, is not so strong as that made from hemp. We took a *chota hagree*, a little breakfast, with the obliging superintendent, and arrived in town again about nine o'clock, at the regular breakfast hour.

FRANK VINCENT, JUN.
The Land of the White Elephant (1873)

1873

Who would be a Snake?

E.K. Laird was a Scot travelling alone round the world, simply for
pleasure. He stayed a fortnight in Singapore with a family friend and
recorded his experiences in a daily journal which he later published.

Thursday, 28th. – Reached Singapore at seven p.m., after a good run. It
is 700 miles from Cheribon, and we came in sixty-two hours. The heat
in the middle of the day was worthy of the Red Sea; however, it became
cooler in the afternoon. I took a trap on landing, and drove straight to
Captain C＿＿, who has a charming house, with fine view of town
and harbour. . . . My cabman as usual wanted double his fare, and I was
just going to give him something extra, when out rushed the Captain,
using language that only a skipper can, and wound up by saying in a
loud voice "For I am a Liverpool man." This last threat at the cabby
completely non-plussed him, as being a Kling I do not suppose he understood a word of it. However, it ended in his getting a dollar.

Friday, 29th. – Busy all morning buying various things; amongst others
buttons, for the Madras fellows who are the Dobies wash the clothes in
a most dreadful manner; one fancies that your carpets are being beaten,
but it is only your unfortunate clothes being violently dashed against a
board, in consequence the buttons are smashed, and your shirts, &c.,
have large gaps in them. . . . Captain C＿＿ took me a long drive yesterday all round the neighbourhood; but now I must stop as it is time to
think of dressing, and besides some freshly-gathered mangosteens, the
queen of fruits, have just come in. . . .

Saturday, 30th. – Captain C＿＿ very kindly gave me permission to
ask C＿＿ up here to lunch, as there is such a perfect all-round view.
We then drove to the Botanical Gardens. In the evening there were four
ladies and their husbands to dinner. Singapore lies low; but there are
numerous hills about, and on them gentlemen build their houses. The
island is covered with jungle, with the feathery palm sticking up – in

fact, from this house as far as one can see, except the side where the town lies, a sombre green covers universal nature; it does not appear to be much cultivated, and I fancy that vegetables come from the mainland. Singapore owes its importance to – first of all, being a free port, and ships and schooners come here from all parts to unload their cargoes in preference to going to Java, so the protective policy of the Dutch has done some good; then it is a great coaling place for steamers *en route* to China and Japan – in fact it is a second Gibraltar without the fortifications; but there are so many islands all around, and the passage so narrow and water so shallow, that a few torpedoes and small gunboats would be efficient protection. There is a regiment here and a few artillery men, and a fort overlooking the town; but I should think that it must only be for keeping the natives in awe – for, as the town lies directly underneath, if they were to attempt to fire out to sea it would bring the fire of an attacking squadron on the city. . . .

Monday, September 1st. . . . I saw a boa-constrictor brought into the town to-day, twenty five feet long; it was caught only six miles from here and was killed whilst in a state of stupor, having just demolished a large sow weighing about two hundred pounds. The limbs and bones of the pig were broken, but the skin was not much damaged, so it was cut out and was sold for food to the "Heathen Chinee," who also bought the flesh of the boa (which they consider a delicacy), at forty cents the pound. The skin was preserved; it was the largest ever found here; it is not pleasant to think that there are such customers near at hand. I only weigh 118 lbs., so I would have been a mere pastime for it; but I flatter myself that I would have been somewhat angular and more difficult of digestion; however, if he had, as they always do, covered me with saliva I dare say I would have glided down easily enough – what a curious idea; I suppose the boa would have waited in a state of stupor until the pig had rotted or dissolved, because it could not move when caught. *I am told* that one was once found with the head of a deer sticking out of its mouth, as the horns were rather too much of a good thing, even for a boa; so it would have slept until the horns gradually dropped off from decay. Who would be a snake?. . .

Wednesday, 3rd. – Spent the morning quietly. In the afternoon drove to Botanical Gardens and heard the band play. The first battalion of the 10th are here, and very good music it was. What would I give now for an opera? however, the more I travel the more I am convinced that I like to live in a civilised manner, and after the feeding in Java it really is quite delightful to feel that one is in a place where a chop can be done plain, and not swimming in cocoa-nut oil. Just as I was going out to-day by the front door a snake about three feet long was on the door-step. It was black in colour and yellow underneath; it wriggled away at about the rate of five miles an hour, at least I know we had to go at a jog-trot to keep up with it. It was killed by one of the servants. It is poisonous I believe, but fortunately I do not fancy that they approve of going upstairs. It was a whip-snake. The tree that I have mentioned as spreading out its leaves in the shape of a fan is called the Traveller's Palm; I did not know the reason why until yesterday; I thought it might be from its beauty. Imagine leaves say six feet in length and one foot across spreading out in the shape of a fan; but it turns out that where the leaf joins on to the stem there is a groove, and in this the rain water collects, and if you make an incision into the stalk of the leaf it flows out, hence the name; and although there has not been rain for some time, out of one of the trees we got a glassful yesterday. It was of course pure rain water and very soft to the taste. As soon as the leaves become perfectly dry they drop off. . . .

Thursday, 4th. – Spent morning in procuring money and taking ticket for "Bokhara." Lunched with Mr. S _____ . . . He afterwards took me over his godowns. I had up to this time a very vague idea of what gambier was; it is the leaves of a shrub boiled down, and pressed till it becomes a brown sticky mass; it is used for tanning hides, also for medicine. I believe it is very stringent. The natives here mix it with betel-nut and cære, and chew it like a quid of tobacco. The Malays have of course to invent words for several things – for instance, ice and telegraph wire; the former they call "stone water," and the latter "speaking rope." Both these are rather good. I do not know the Malay for them, but this is their equivalent in English. The sun they call "eye of day" – also pretty. . . .

Friday, 5th. – Lunched at Club as usual. In evening there were five or six people at dinner. We had some Shanghai mutton, which is considered a great delicacy in these parts.

Saturday, 6th. – "Bokhara" arrived last evening, so that I suppose we will be off Sunday. Packed up and went to the band in the evening. Young B_____ lunched with me at Emerson's, the luncheon place of Singapore. . . .

Sunday, 7th. – Left at twelve. Had heavy squalls of rain, and are not going much more than nine knots. It is 380 miles to Penang. We are coasting along the Peninsula, and can see Sumatra. I have a large cabin to myself, as there are only about twenty passengers. All the best cabins forward are filled with tea, so that if there are many passengers they have to put three or four in one cabin. . . . Very warm and close. I was sorry to leave Captain C____, as he has been most civil; but glad to depart from Singapore, where, without exaggeration, I may say that I have hardly once had a perfectly dry stitch of clothing on for the whole time, except early morning, as, although the thermometer rarely rises above 85, still it is hardly ever below it. But it is considered a healthy place for the East, as although the Europeans look pale they do not have fevers, &c. Cholera has been for some time at Singapore, and if it had not been for the latter I might have visited Borneo, but I think it better to leave the Malay Archipelago.

E.K. LAIRD
The Rambles of a Globe Trotter (1875)

1875

Human Sacrifice

> Many public works in Singapore were carried out by convict labour
> imported from India, and both John McNair and W.D. Bayliss were
> involved in their supervision. Here they describe a recurring problem
> associated with construction work in Singapore.

These convicts from India . . . being wholly different in their habits,
customs, and language from the Chinese who formed the bulk of the
town population, it is not to be wondered at that the Chinese felt themselves estranged from them, and kept themselves ever aloof. There were,
however, some Chinese of the lowest class who sought to embroil themselves with them, so as to bring the convicts into trouble, but the convicts always avoided a quarrel. They therefore sought other means, and
in 1852 they gave out and placarded over the town that the Governor
and all the Europeans had left worshipping in St. Andrew's Church,
owing to the number of evil spirits there, and had gone to worship in
the Court House, and that in order to appease the spirits the Governor
required thirty heads, and had ordered the convicts to waylay people at
night and kill them.

These placards created quite a panic in the place, so that people were
for some days afraid to leave their houses after dark. In order to allay
the fears of the people the Governor issued a proclamation saying that
St. Andrew's Church had been struck by lightning and was unsafe
(which was the fact), and he called upon the people not to believe the
reports of evil men. Moreover, he offered a reward of $500 for the dis-
covery of any person propagating such reports. This had no effect however, so the leading Chinese merchants were called upon to address their
countrymen, which they did in a long appeal, assuring them of the bene-
volence of the Christian Government, and urging them to have no fear
and not believe in foolish reports. In two days the fears of the Chinese
population were thus dispelled. In 1875 a similar "head scare" occurred

during the construction of the "puddle trench" for the new impounding reservoir. This was a work of considerable difficulty, and some superstitious natives circulated a report that it could not be done without "human sacrifice," and that the Government were looking for "heads" to put into the trench, and the alarm for days was so great that people would not pass along Thompson's Road adjoining the reservoir after dark; and even the "dhobies," or washer-men, in the stream adjoining the puddle trench, hastened into town before dusk. Similar so called "head scares" have occurred in Singapore up to even the present time. It is not easy to define what has led to this superstition in the native mind, and it is made more complicated from the fact that it is shared alike by Chinese and natives of India.

J.F.A. MCNAIR & W.D. BAYLISS
Prisoners their own Warders (1899)

1877

Little Short of Slavery

When William Pickering arrived in Singapore he found himself to be "the only European officer ever in the service of the Straits Settlements who could speak Chinese". Initially he was employed as Chinese Interpreter but after the events described below, new laws were introduced and Pickering became the first Protector of Chinese.

This morning about 10.20 a report came to the Police Office that there was a riot in Market Street, to which place Major Dunlop and I hurried; at the junction of Market Street and Boat Quay, we found a large crowd looking towards the other side of the water in the direction of the "Red Lamps." Some respectable Chinese told us that the row was because some Sinkehs refused to be taken on board a vessel; we went on towards the Public Offices and on reaching the Square, met two Chinese bringing four or five Sinkehs along, and one of them held a Sinkeh by the tail, whom he was forcing to accompany him; all these were given in charge to a Policeman to take to the Central Station.

On our arrival at the Public Offices we found a crowd, but all disturbances was over, we were told that 20 or 30 Chinese had been arrested, and that several had been severely beaten; we returned to the Central Station and found more than 20 Sinkehs some of whom were suffering from wounds on the head, legs, and face; one was brought in insensible, in which state he continued some time and was eventually sent to Hospital. After their wounds were dressed, their names were taken down, and we discovered that they had only been landed a day or two from Hainam Junks, and after being shut up closely in a house in Teluk Ayer, they had been disposed of to the Chinese Agent of a Dutch gentleman for $35 dollars each to work in Sumatra.

These men are for the most part natives of places far in the interior of China. They all cried out most piteously for protection; as they declared they had been induced to leave their homes by promises to the effect that they should be brought to Singapore only, and receive good wages as carpenters, sawyers, brickmakers, &c, and that after paying a very low sum for their passages, they would soon save money enough to send to their friends or to return home with. They had heard that instead of this they were being sent to work in the tin-mines of another country, so refused to go on board the Tongkangs. On this the Emigration Agents or Khehtows had threatened them with punishment by our officials, and had beaten them. . . .

During the afternoon the statements of . . . some of the sinkehs were taken down, of which I append copies, and I think these plainly show that the system, under which at least Hainam junks bring down Chinese Immigrants, is little short of slavery.

STATEMENTS

Chew-Ah-Nyee, – I come from the prefecture of Kow-Chew-foo, and am a School-master. I was engaged in teaching, when about the 24th of the 11th moon, Chiang-See and Kuai-leong told me that they could get me plenty of work at Singapore as a clerk, and that wages here were very good; I believed them, and was put on board a junk and brought to this place, where I was sold to a shop, chop "Hiap-tye." We came on shore on the 2nd of the 1st moon, there were 90 men from my district, the strong men were sent to saw-yards I believe, but I was sold as a "little pig" being weak. This morning I was being taken to a boat with many others, I don't know where they were taking us to, but we heard that the place is 11 or 12 days' sail from this, and that we had to work in tin-mines; of course we refused to go to another country, as we had understood Singapore to be our destination, and I can't work as a miner. On our way to the boat we refused to proceed, so the Khehtows struck us and threatened us with the Mandarins; they did call the Government Officials who struck me and my companions, and we were afterwards brought here. Chiang-see and Kuai-leong paid my passage here, but it was on the understanding, that when I got employment at Singapore, I should repay them. I never thought of being sold to work in tin-mines. All the money I have received is $1 in copper to buy clothes with.

Leong-ship-sam (an old man), – I am a Kwang-si man from Kwei-lin-foo and am a carpenter, but can do other work also. Kiet-ug came to me in the 11th moon and said if you will come with me to Singapore, I will show you how to make lots of money, with which you can keep your wife and family. I followed him bringing with me a few clothes and 1,000 cash ($1) and was 10 days in arriving at Hoi-Low where I with seventeen others from neighbourhood was put on board a Hainam junk. I don't know what the passage money was, but Kiet-ug said it would be very cheap and that we could soon get money by work at Singapore to repay it. We arrived here on the 29th of the 12th moon (11th February) and were landed on the 2nd of the 1st moon (14th February) at night, after our evening rice. We were taken to a house upstairs and not allowed to come down till this morning; we were within two or three doors and not allowed even a smoke, we were kept in ignorance and could not see the sky, until to-day, when we were told that we must work in some tin mines. This morning they hurried us over our meal, and said we must go away; I had saved a few cash which I gave a man to buy tobacco for me. I and fourteen others were sent on board a boat, and if the gentlemen had not come and delivered me, I should have been stolen away in ignorance. I wanted to come to this place but don't wish to go elsewhere. They gave us altogether $2 this morning to buy clothes with, but would not give us a chance to spend it, as they pushed us down towards the boat.

Lew-ship-yit, – I am neighbour of Leong-ship-sam and am a labourer; Kiet-ug induced me to leave China by saying, "look how poor you are here, if you follow me, I can take you to Singapore, where you will get such good employment, that very soon you will pay the small amount of passage-money required and will save more than $50 or $60 per year." On arriving here we were taken to a shop upstairs and were barred up, only having a very little rice and saltfish; we could not go out to the stool, or have a smoke. I don't much complain about food, as long as I can get some work to make money, but we were shut up and not allowed to know what was being done with us. This morning Chiang See gave us two dollars but he took 95 cents for a jacket, 55 cents for a pair of trousers and kept from me the balance. I was being taken on board a boat with a lot of others, and if any refused to go they were beaten by the Khehtows, there was a row and I got a blow during the struggle. I don't wish to go past Singapore, this is the place I agreed to come to.

––––––––

Major Dunlop and I went to inspect the house . . . in Teluk Ayer, where the coolies had been confined. We found the place at the very top of the house, and "not fit" as the Major said, "to keep pigs in," many men might be confined here without notice, and everything confirmed the statements of the Sinkehs.

It must be confessed that such a state of things as the above cannot be called creditable to any government, but especially to one like ours, supposed to be based on principles of justice and freedom; no doubt a great deal of the evil is the result of our over-anxiety not to interfere with the liberty of the Chinaman, and to abstain from vexatious regulations, which might impede free immigration of labour into these colonies. I would however humbly suggest that some steps be taken immediately to protect in some way the newly arrived Chinese from extortion and oppression. . . .

W.A. PICKERING
"Report by Mr. Pickering on Kidnapping Senkehs"
Paper laid before the Legislative Council, February 1877

1877

Hot Dusty Town

Annie Brassey and family sailed round the world in their private schooner "Sunbeam" on a voyage that lasted forty-six weeks. Her husband Thomas, a British politician with an interest in naval affairs, was later to become Governor of the Australian colony of Victoria. The "Sunbeam" made a brief stop at Singapore to take on coal and other supplies.

Saturday, March 17th. – We were off Singapore during the night. At 5 a.m. the pilot came on board and took us into Tangong Pagar to coal alongside the wharf. We left the ship as soon as possible, and in about an hour we had taken forty-three tons of coal on board and nearly twenty tons of water. The work was rapidly performed by coolies. It was a great disappointment to be told by the harbour-master that the Governor of the Straits Settlements and Lady Jervoise were to leave at eleven o'clock for Johore. We determined to go straight to the Government House and make a morning call at the unearthly hour of 8 a.m. The drive from the wharf was full of beauty, novelty, and interest. We had not landed so near the line before, and the most tropical of tropical plants, trees, flowers, and ferns, were here to be seen, growing by the roadside on every bank and dust-heap.

The natives, Malays, are a fine-looking, copper-coloured race, wearing bright-coloured sarongs and turbans. There are many Indians, too, from Madras, almost black, and swathed in the most graceful white muslin garments, when they are not too hard at work to wear anything at all. The young women are very good-looking. They wear not only one but several rings, and metal ornaments in their noses, and a profusion of metal bangles on their arms and legs, which jingle and jangle as they move.

The town of Singapore itself is not imposing, its streets, or rather roads of wooden huts and stone houses, being mixed together indiscriminately. Government House is on the outskirts of the city, in the midst of a beautiful park. The House itself is large and handsome, with suites of lofty rooms, shaded by wide verandahs, full of ferns and palms. We found the Governor and his family did not start until 11.30, and they kindly begged us to return to breakfast at half-past nine, which we did. Before finally leaving, Sir William Jervoise sent for the Colonial Secretary, and asked him to look after us in his absence. He turned out to be an old schoolfellow and college friend of Tom's at Rugby and Oxford; so the meeting was a very pleasant one. As soon as the Governor and his suite had set off for Johore we went down into the hot dusty town to get our letters, parcels, and papers, and to look at the shops.

The north-east monsoon still blows fresh and strong, but it was nevertheless terribly hot in the streets, and we were very glad to return to the cool, shady rooms at Government House, where we thoroughly appreciated the delights of the punkah.

There are very few European servants here, and they all have their own peons to wait on them, and carry an umbrella over them when they drive the carriage or go for a walk on their own account. Even the private soldier in Singapore has a punkah pulled over his bed at night. It is quite a sight to meet all the coolies leaving barracks at 5 a.m., when they have done punkah-pulling.

At four o'clock Mr. Douglas called to take us for a drive. We went first to the Botanical Gardens, and saw sago-palms and all sorts of tropical produce flourishing in perfection. There were many beautiful birds and beasts ... The cages were large, and the enclosures in front full of Cape jasmine bushes (covered with buds) for the birds to peck at and eat. From the gardens we went for a drive through the pretty villas that surround Singapore in every direction. It was dark when we returned to dine at Government House.

Sunday, March 18th. – At six o'clock this morning Mabelle and I went ashore with the steward and the comprador to the market. It is a nice, clean, octagonal building, well supplied with vegetables and curious fruits. The latter are mostly brought from the other islands, as this is the worst season of the year in Singapore for fruit. We tasted many fruits new to us – delicious mangosteens, lacas, and other fruits whose names I could not ascertain. Lastly, we tried a durian, *the* fruit of the East, as it is called by people who live here; and having got over the first horror of the onion-like odour, we found it by no means bad.

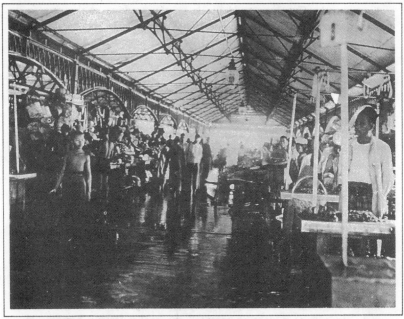

INSIDE MARKET

The fish market is the cleanest, and best arranged, and sweetest smelling that I ever went through. It is situated on a sort of open platform, under a thick thatched roof, built out over the sea, so that all the refuse is easily disposed of and washed away by the tide. From the platform on which it stands, two long jetties run out into the sea, so that large fishing boats can come alongside and discharge their cargoes at the door of the market.

The poultry market is a curious place. On account of the intense heat everything is brought alive to the market, and the quacking, cackling, gobbling, and crowing that go on are really marvellous. The whole street is alive with birds in baskets, cages, and coops, or tied by the leg and thrown down anyhow.... They are all very tame and very cheap; and some of the scarlet lories, looking like a flame of fire, chatter in the most amusing way. I have a cage full of tiny parrots not bigger than bullfinches, of a dark green colour, with dark red throats and blue heads, yellow marks on the back, and red and yellow tails. Having bought these, everybody seemed to think that I wanted an unlimited supply of birds, and soon we were surrounded by a chattering crowd, all with parrots in their hands and on their shoulders. It was a very amusing sight, though rather noisy, and the competition reduced the prices very much. Parrakeets ranged from twelve to thirty cents apiece, talking parrots and cockatoos from one to five dollars. At last the vendors became so energetic that I was glad to get into the gharry again, and drive away to a flower shop, where we bought some gardenias for one penny a dozen, beautifully fresh and fragrant, but with painfully short stalks.

Towards the end of the south-west monsoon, little native open boats arrive from the islands 500 to 1,500 miles to the south-eastward of Singapore. Each has one little tripod mast. The whole family live on board. The sides of the boat cannot be seen for the multitudes of cockatoos, parrots, parrakeets, and birds of all sorts, fastened on little perches, with very short strings attached to them. The decks are covered with sandal-wood. The holds are full of spice, shells, feathers, and South Sea pearl shells. With this cargo they creep from island to island, and from creek to creek, before the monsoon, till they reach their destination. They stay a month or six weeks, change their goods for iron, nails, a certain amount of pale green or Indian red thread for weaving, and some pieces of Manchester cotton. They then go back with the north-east monsoon, selling their goods at the various islands on their homeward route. There are many Dutch ports nearer than Singapore, but they are over-regulated, and preference is given to the free English port, where the simple natives can do as they like so long as they do not transgress the laws.

MRS. BRASSEY
A Voyage in the "Sunbeam" (1878)

1877

A Fortune Teller

After thirty-five years in the East, including service with the Bengal Marine, J.D. Vaughan set up a law office in Singapore. He became popular in local amateur theatricals and was considered a talented singer. Tragically, when returning from a visit to Perak, Vaughan disappeared while on board ship – a fate not predicted here by his Chinese fortune teller.

In Singapore the Tay Chews have two [Chinese temples] in Phillip Street within the same enclosure, dedicated to the idol "Gwan Thien Siang Tey," and several about the country called by the same name. The buildings in Town are very old and much neglected, there are no priests attached to them; and are in charge of a Kling policeman. In each building sits a Chinese ready to sell incense sticks, and sacrificial papers to worshippers. A fortune teller has a stall there also. He sits at a table with a tray before him in which are placed a number of folded papers. He also has a glass slate, indian ink, and hair pencils at hand. For a few cents he told the writer his fortune, and appeared highly amused at a European favoring him. One of the folded papers was selected and opened. On it appeared a Chinese character. This the fortune teller copied on the slate and surrounded it with a number of strokes which appeared to resemble portions of Chinese letters. He then muttered a formula and ever and anon completed the half written characters; or added a stroke here and a stroke there until his incantations were complete. By this time the letters were finished and assumed the shape of well-known Chinese characters. He then commenced repeating the result in a loud tone. Till the end of the current year 1877 the writer was to be unfortunate but after that he would be lucky and grow rich. That his lines were cast in pleasant places and he ought to be thankful. He then smiled complacently and said the oracle had finished. The writer moved on making way for a sturdy Tay Chew cooly who appeared highly satisfied with the result and seemed anxious to obtain as favorable a fortune told for himself. The Chinese have great confidence in these fortune tellers, and scarcely undertake an event in life without consulting them or the idols.

In each temple were dingy pictures and images placed in niches far back with stands and vases full of artificial flowers and burnt out incense sticks, with numerous lanterns and glass lamps hung from the rafters, or placed on the stands. Behind the temples are a few rooms filled with portions of small carriages and sedan chairs which are put together and used in processions. In each temple are stone tablets let into the wall perpetuating the names of the original sub-scribers. In the front of the temples is a large flagged square surrounded by a high wall, in which temporary stages are erected for theatrical performances; when of course the place is crowded by worshippers, who are attracted more by them, than the service of the gods. Chinese gods appear to be particularly fond of the drama. The wise say that these performances are often given to screen gamblers who play in adjoining houses, whilst the attention of the police is attracted to the crowd before the theatre. Chinese worship consists in lighting incense sticks and placing them before the idols; burning sacrificial paper and bowing two or three times, or kowtowing, before the images. Heart worship there is none. Except at festivals there is no worship of any kind conducted in these Tay Chew temples. In the temples in the country live one or two men who sweep them daily and make a living by selling incense sticks, sacrificial paper and candles to worshippers; besides pocketing the alms that are bestowed upon them. Some of these men get as much as thirty dollars a month; and others grow rich; these posts are coveted and strenuous efforts are made to get them. In each of the Town temples are staves placed in racks with symbols resembling the sun, moon, swords and other things placed on their tips conveying doubtless a deep signification to the learned; but certainly none to the common herd, who have never been able to afford the writer the slightest information on the subject. There is no indication of the Budhist religion in these temples. No idols or pictures of Hindu deities are in them. It is un-doubted that the Chinese in the Straits do not pretend to worship any idol or picture representing God, but only those of deified hu-man beings who are supposed to intercede with the Almighty for mortals below. . . .

In Singapore on the 26th of the 10th month the Tay Chews carry their idol in procession from their cemetery at Tanglin to their temple in Phillip Street to see the theatricals held there in his honor. The idol is kept there till the 11th moon when it is carried back with the same ceremony. The Hokiens have a similar procession once in three years; the idol at their cemetery on the New Harbour road is carried in procession through the parts of the Town chiefly inhabited by Hokiens to the great Hokien temple in Teluk Ayer Street, where it is left for a short period and then taken back to its own temple at the cemetery. Their procession is gorgeous in the extreme and costs the Hokien community a large sum of money. It is accompanied by coolies bearing flags, umbrellas, symbols, sedan chairs, and bands of music making the most horrible din. One wonders that such practical people, whose whole time is devoted to the acquisition of wealth should waste their money upon such absurdities; yet they can be scarcely ridiculed when we think of the absurd processions that occur in civilized London. The writer witnessed the Lord Mayor's show in 1874 and was much struck by its strong resemblance to the Chinese processions in the Straits.

J.D. VAUGHAN
The Manners and Customs of the
Chinese of the Straits Settlements (1879)

1878

How Odd Everything Looked

For well over two years William Hornaday travelled through India, Ceylon, Borneo and the Malay Peninsula. His job was to collect natural history specimens for Professor Ward of Rochester, New York, whose Natural Science Establishment was world famous. Hornaday, who was later to become Chief Taxidermist at the U.S. National Museum, spent a week in Singapore.

Entering Singapore by way of New Harbor is like getting into a house through the scullery window. One's first impressions of the town are associated with coal-dust, mud, stagnant water, and mean buildings, and I found it required quite an effort to shake them off. This back-door entrance is by no means fair to Singapore, for under its baleful influence the traveller is apt to go away (by the next steamer usually) with a low estimate of the city, every way considered.

For the first stage out from New Harbor, the road is built through a muddy and dismal mangrove swamp. Here and there we pass a group of dingy and weather-beaten Malay houses standing on posts over the soft and slimy mud, or perhaps over a thin sheet of murky water. Delightful situation, truly, for the habitations of civilized human beings. Monkeys would choose much better. A Malay prefers to build over water; and, failing that, he builds over the softest mud he can find, usually on the bank of a river or lagoon. His house is quite in keeping with its location. The roof is made of palm leaves, and very often the walls also. The windows are mere slits across the wall near the floor, with clumsy wooden bars across; there is not a speck of paint or whitewash or colored paper visible anywhere, and the whole structure reminds one of an old crow's nest.

Farther on, we emerge from the swamp and pass a Chinese Joss house and cemetery on a hill-side, beyond which we have for a mile, on our right hand, a solid row of Chinese shops and dwellings, and

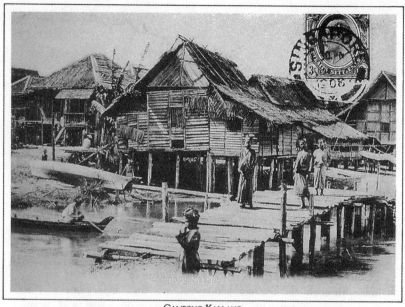

CAMPONG KALLANG

on the other side of the road, a creek flowing mud and slime instead of water. Talk of malaria! It could be cut in that creek, in blocks a foot square, like ice in the Hudson. And the worst of it is that creek stinks – pardon, I mean sticks – by us until we are well into the city itself.

How odd the Chinese shops look with their huge red lanterns, wonderful signs, and flaming inscriptions in black on red paper pasted on the door-posts, lintels, and window-casings. How fat and sleek and hearty-looking are all the Chinese men and women, and how plump and saucy-looking are all their children. I am sure the Chinese are more fleshy, man for man, than any other people in the world.

Rattling on we go. Here are Chinamen smoking big stems of bamboo, large enough for hitching-posts; here is one having his pig-tail combed and his head shaved as he sits smoking unconcernedly on a bench. We pass four Chinamen with a huge and clumsy coffin upon a cart in which there will soon be a fifth, please heaven. Here is a Malay woman combing her hair in a doorway, and here . . . are three shops kept by Tamils, or Klings, as they call them here.

108

How odd everything looks. The houses are all two stories high, with part of the lower story cut out to give a dry passage way, and the overhanging upper portion supported by huge square pillars of masonry.

Aha! The sailors' quarter, it would seem, if we may judge by the tavern signs. One announces, quite regardless of space,

THEMANONTHELOOKOUT,

and displays the portly figure of a Jack tar holding a small Krupp cannon up to his eye, while he squints horribly into the muzzle. Another sign in base imitation of the former proclaims,

THEMANATTHEWHEEL;

and another, the best painted of them all, sets forth, in beautiful letters but homicidal orthography,

THE SILVER ANKER.

Still another proclaims

THE ORIGINAL MADRAS BOB,

which is equivalent to the assertion that there are spurious Madras Bobs about, and "all others are base imitations, unless stamped by our trade mark, and liable to be prosecuted according to law." Verily human nature seems to be very much the same in Singapore as in Rochester.

The streets are wide, the shops are trim and orderly, and apparently filled to overflowing with their respective wares. What fine times we shall have loafing about these queer streets, and poking our nose into everything that is new!

Just now, however, it is pouring rain, so we rattle on through the Chinese bazaars, across an iron bridge, spanning a sort of inner harbor for lighters and small boats (Singapore River), and, without having passed a single European house or shop, we alight at a hotel just at the foot of Fort-Canning-on-the-hill.

Singapore is certainly the handiest city I ever saw, as well planned and carefully executed as though built entirely by one man. It is like a big desk, full of drawers and pigeon-holes, where everything has its place, and can always be found in it. For instance, around the esplanade you find the European hotels – and bad enough they are, too; around Commercial Square, packed closely together, are all the shipping offices, warehouses, and shops of the European merchants; and along Boat Quay are all the ship chandlers. Near by, you will find a dozen large Chinese medicine shops, a dozen cloth shops, a dozen tin shops, and similar clusters of shops kept by blacksmiths, tailors, and carpenters, others for the sale of fruit, vegetables, grain, "notions," and so on to the end of the chapter. All the washerwomen congregate on a five-acre lawn called Dhobi Green, at one side of which runs a stream of water, and there you will see the white shirts, trowsers, and pajamas of His Excellency, perhaps, hanging in ignominious proximity to and on a level with yours. By some means or other, even the Joss houses, like birds of a feather, have flocked together at one side of the town. Owing to this peculiar grouping of the different trades, one can do more business in less time in Singapore than in any other town in the world.

Architecturally considered, Singapore has little to boast of except solidity and uniformity. With but few exceptions the buildings are all Chinese, and perfectly innocent of style. It is a two-story town throughout, solidly built of brick, plastered over, and painted a very pale blue or light yellow. There is a remarkable scarcity of the tumbledown, drunk, and disreputable old buildings so essential to the integrity of all other large cities. Some of the Chinese shops and dwellings of the rich merchants are quite elaborately ornamented on the front with fancy tile and brick work, figures of apocryphal dragons and Chinese lions in high relief, and surrounded by beautifully kept gardens of tropical plants and shrubs. All of these impart a tasty and luxuriant air to the streets. The wealthy Chinamen take very kindly to European luxuries of all kinds except in matters of dress. They are lavish in the use of fine furniture, wines, and food, and their turnouts are really dazzling with their fine open carriages, matched horses, elegant harnesses, and liveried servants, though in dress they draw the line at the white stiff hat of English make. Their dress is cool and roomy, made of white silk or linen, and they wear no jewelry whatever.

The population of Singapore (about one hundred thousand) is a sort of *omnium gatherum* from the various over-crowded countries of Southern Asia generally. The Chinese are by far the most numerous, the most thrifty and enterprising, and the most satisfactory to deal with. The Malays come next, and after them the Tamils from Southern India and Ceylon. The population includes a goodly sprinkling of Portuguese half-castes, a few Javanese, a few Siamese, and of

Europeans, a mixture of English, Dutch, Germans, French, Swiss, and last but not least, three Americans, our consul and his daughters.

Of the social life of Singapore I know nothing; but from what I was told, I judge it is not at all different from other British colonies. There are the usual balls and dinner parties, and the usual number of grades in society, each of which knows its station to a line and never ventures beyond it. To an American it seems extremely silly for wholesale merchants and their clerks to hold themselves, socially, above the retail merchants and their clerks, regardless of the amount of business they do, and their moral and intellectual standing. For my part, I have no patience with society's nonsensical standards, in accordance with which a man's business or profession is everything, and he himself is nothing. Thank God for America, where every man stands on his merits, if he has any.

The hotels of Singapore are all bad, and life in them is exceedingly dull. The liquor consumed in them, and the drunken men one sees almost daily, keep the abstemious traveller in a state of perpetual disgust. The extent to which intoxicating liquors of all kinds are drunk in the East Indies is simply appalling. The drinking habit is so universal, that, as a general thing, when you go to call on an acquaintance at his house, or to visit a stranger in company with other friends, the greeting is, "What will you have to drink?" If you say you do not drink, or do not wish anything, you are urged most urgently to "take *something*," until it becomes positively disagreeable; and really the easiest way is to compromise by taking a glass of their beastly lemonade or abominable soda. Furthermore, when your new acquaintances, or old ones either, for that matter, call upon you at your hotel for half an hour's chat, you are expected to order drinks for the crowd, until the crowd is full of whatever it likes best. To omit this feature is to give positive offence in some cases, and even at the best to send your visitors away saying that you are uncivil and not worthy the acquaintance of gentlemen.

WILLIAM T. HORNADAY
Two Years in the Jungle (1885)

1879

Fashion

The American philanthropist, Andrew Carnegie, who made his fortune in iron and steel, sailed westwards from San Francisco on his voyage round the world. In Singapore he seemed particularly interested in the subject of clothes – an interest that could perhaps be traced to his humble beginnings as a weaver's assistant in a cotton factory.

SINGAPORE, Saturday, January 4.

We reached Singapore at dusk. The drive through the town was a curious one. Nowhere else can such a mixture of races be seen, and each nationality was enjoying itself in its own peculiar fashion – all except the Chinese, who were, as usual, hard at work in their little dens. No recreation for this people. Work, work, work! They never play, never smile, but plod away, from early morning until late at night....

We saw in Singapore our first lot of Hindoos, moving about the streets like ghosts, wrapped in webs of thin white cotton cloth, which scissors, needle, or thread have never defiled. The cloth must remain just as it came from the loom; no hat, no shoes, their foreheads chalked, or painted in red with the stamp of the god they worship and the caste to which they belong. They are a small, slight race, with fine, delicate features....

We were driven one day, by the major and Miss Studer, some ten or twelve miles in the interior, passing through groves of cocoa and betel-nut trees, both in full bearing, to a tapioca plantation, where we saw many trees and plants new to us – the fan and sago palms and many other varieties, bananas, nutmeg trees, bread fruit, durion, gutta-percha trees and others. We also saw the indigo plant under cultivation, and passed through fields of the sensitive plant as we walked about, while pine-apples were everywhere. We are in a new world of vegetation here, within a degree of the Equator; but, rich as it is, there is still a feeling of disappointment because it is all green – no bright hues, no coloring, such as gives Florida its charm, or lends to an American forest in autumn its unrivalled glory! It is always summer, and the moisture of the tropics keeps everything green.

. . . This drive gave us an excellent opportunity of seeing just how the people live in the country. Dress is confined to the rag worn about the loins, except that the women wear in addition a small cloth over their shoulders. The children wear nothing whatever, but we saw none that were not ornamented by cheap jewelry in the most extraordinary manner.

The subject of clothes, as we all know from the days of "Sartor Resartus," lies very closely at the roots of civilization. I think every thoughtful person must admit that here the Heathen Chinee shows that he has reached the best solution of that annoying question. The every-day dress of the Chinaman is to-day just what it was thousands of years ago. As there is no going out or coming in of fashion, he wears his clothes till they can be worn no longer. The heavy overcoats which distress Americans and are a weight even to the Englishman, our celestial friend escapes by having three or four light coats all of one pattern and weight. It is a one, two, or a three-coat day, according to temperature. Again and above all he escapes the horrid starch entirely, neither shirts nor collars nor cuffs, sometimes like thin sheets of iron, irritating his skin.

Vandy and I seriously resolved to-day that we would never again tolerate a starched thing about us; no matter what others did, we would discard the vile custom and be free. . . .

Vandy and I when in the East reduced the time for bathing and dressing in the morning to seven minutes. Of course, we have long since given up the folly of shaving. How one envies the man of the East who has but four articles to slip on, and no pins required: socks and low shoes (no lacing), one; breeches, two; undershirt, three; coat, four; and there he is, ready for breakfast. The coat buttons close to the chin, and has a small upright collar, and a watch-pocket outside; no cuffs, collars or neckties. Why does not some born reformer of our sex devote his life to giving his fellow man such additional happiness in life? Hundreds waste their energies upon objects which, if accomplished, would not be half as fruitful. . . .

The climate of Singapore, as of all places so near the Equator,

113

would be intolerable but for the dense clouds which obscure the sun and save us from its fierce rays; but occasionally it breaks through for a few minutes, and we are in a bath of perspiration before we know it. No one can estimate the difference in the power of the sun here as compared with it in New York. Straw hats afford no protection whatever; we are compelled to wear thick white helmets of pith, and use a white umbrella lined with green cloth, and yet can walk only a few steps when the sun is not hid without feeling that we must seek the shade. The horses are unable to go more than ten miles in twenty-four hours, and our carriage and pair are hired with the understanding that this is not to be exceeded. Nothing could exist near the line if the intense heat did not cause evaporation upon a gigantic scale. The clouds so formed are driven upward by the streams of colder air from both sides, condensation then takes place, and showers fall every few hours in the region of Singapore.

ANDREW CARNEGIE
Round the World (1888)

1879

A Very Agreeable Guest

Colonel A.E.H. Anson, Lieutenant-Governor at Penang, came to Singapore to take charge for a year until the arrival of the new Governor, Sir Frederick Weld. Anson had something of a reputation among his superiors in London for lack of judgement, and his arrangements for General Grant's visit to Singapore were perhaps not untypical. Nevertheless he was later promoted to Major-General and subsequently knighted.

Early in 1879, I received intimation that General Grant, the ex-President of the United States of America, would shortly visit the colony. I therefore sent to the American Consul, and invited him to come and see me at Government House; and when he came, I asked him what General Grant's position was, as I wished to know how to receive him. He said he is not this, nor that, nor the other, mentioning different appointments; but he is a very great man. Not being able to obtain any definite information from the Consul, I telegraphed to the Chief Commissioner at Burmah, where the General had just arrived; and asked how he had been received there. The reply came: "With a military guard of honour and a salute." On this I telegraphed to the Acting Lieutenant-Governor of Penang to receive the General with those honours. However, while the General was at Penang, the English mail passed there, and arriving at Singapore, brought me a dispatch from the Secretary of State for the Colonies, instructing me that in accordance, I understood, with the wishes of the American Government, these honours were not to be accorded to the General. I accordingly gave orders that he should be received on landing, with a guard of the armed police force, and by the principal officers of the Government. This led to his secretary, on landing, remarking to one of the colonial officials, "What, no soldiers here?"

115

On the night of his arrival, I entertained the General, Mrs Grant, and his suite at dinner, and held a reception afterwards; and then gave a ball. I was told that the General objected to making speeches, so at the end of dinner, after proposing the healths of the Queen and the President of the United States, I rose from the table. I was informed afterwards, that the General was much disappointed, as he had prepared a speech for the occasion. I found him a very agreeable and interesting guest. He had visited every crowned head in Europe, and been to India, Burmah, etc., and when chatting in the verandah of an evening, after dinner, I found him very entertaining. I one day said to Mrs Grant, "When you go back to the White House, I suppose you will do so and so." She replied, "Oh yes," and then emphatically remarked, "If he heard me he would knock my head off." Another time, when she had been telling me about all the beautiful things she had bought in Paris, I said, "Why don't you send them to Mrs. Hayes (the President's wife), and ask her to take care of them for you at the White House." She said, "Oh yes, Mrs Hayes is a friend of mine, and would do it for me, but——," and then she made use of the same expression, with the same action, as on the former occasion. There is no doubt she looked to her husband being elected President for the third time. I asked him what he thought of his chance of being so, and he said, "Were the elections going to take place this year, I think I should have a fair chance, but as they do not, I cannot be sure of the stability of public sentiment."

The General was very proud of having commanded a million men in the Civil War of America.

Mrs Grant, in talking of her husband before he became President, used to say, "That was before Ulys was a great man." She told me that while the General was President she had, with him, visited the Mormon City, and interviewed the chief wife of Brigham Young, who, after upholding their marriage system for some time, burst into tears and exclaimed, "It is hell on earth!"

Mrs Grant, in speaking of my aide-de-camp, said, "He's a sweet lad," and he was, for some time afterwards, known by that name in his regiment.

There was, at Singapore, a dear old Chinaman named Whampoa, a general favourite. He was a member of the Legislative Council, and a C.M.G. He had a charming country house and garden. His drawing-rooms were fitted up in Chinese style, with a circle of carved and gilded wood separating one room from the other. His garden . . .

was laid out like the willow-pattern plates, with the summer-house and bridge over the water, which abounded in gold fish, which used to be fed by the visitors. Wishing to entertain General Grant, he invited him to lunch, and me to accompany him. There was a large party, one of which was an American, the only countryman Whampoa could find available at the moment. He was a dentist of a rather inferior social position. As we were driving home together, after the party, General Grant turned to me and said, "Why did Whampoa ask that tooth carpenter to meet me?"

MAJOR-GENERAL SIR ARCHIBALD ANSON
About Others and Myself (1920)

1879

Punkahs Everywhere

One of the outstanding travellers – and travel writers – of the century, Isabella Bird was forty-seven when she visited Singapore. She had just spent several months exploring Japan, and was about to embark on a journey through the Malay States. In between she made a brief stop at Singapore and wrote about it in a letter to her sister in Edinburgh.

I had scarcely finished breakfast at the hotel, a shady, straggling building, much infested by ants, when Mr. Cecil Smith, the Colonial Secretary, and his wife called, full of kind thoughts and plans of furtherance; and a little later a resident, to whom I had not even a letter of introduction, took me and my luggage to his bungalow. All the European houses seem to have very deep verandahs, large, lofty rooms, punkahs everywhere, windows without glass, brick floors, and jalousies and "tatties" (blinds made of grass or finely-split bamboo) to keep out the light and the flies. This equatorial heat is neither as exhausting or depressing as the damp summer heat of Japan, though one does long "to take off one's flesh and sit in one's bones.". . .

As Singapore is a military station, and ships of war hang about constantly, there is a great deal of fluctuating society, and the officials of the Straits Settlements Government are numerous enough to form a large society of their own. Then there is the merchant class, English, German, French, and American; and there is the usual round of gaiety, and of the amusements which make life intolerable. I think that in most of these tropical colonies the ladies exist only on the hope of going "home!" It is a dreary, aimless life for them – scarcely life, only existence. The greatest sign of vitality in Singapore Europeans that I can see is the furious hurry in writing for the mail. To all sorts of claims and invitations, the reply is, "But it's mail day, you know," or, "I'm writing for the mail," or, "I'm awfully behind hand

118

with my letters," or, "I can't stir till the mail's gone!" The hurry is desperate, and even the feeble Englishwomen exert themselves for "friends at home." To judge from the flurry and excitement, and the driving down to the post-office at the last moment, and the commotion in the parboiled community, one would suppose the mail to be an uncertain event occurring once in a year or two, rather than the most regular of weekly fixtures! The incoming mail is also a great event, though its public and commercial news is anticipated by four weeks by the telegraph. . . .

My short visit has been mainly occupied with the day at the Colonial Secretary's Lodge, and in walking and driving through the streets. The city is ablaze with colour and motley with costume. The ruling race does not show to advantage. A pale-skinned man or woman, costumed in our ugly, graceless clothes, reminds one not pleasingly, artistically at least, of our dim, pale islands. Every Oriental costume from the Levant to China floats through the streets – robes of silk, satin, brocade, and white muslin, emphasised by the glitter of "barbaric gold;" and Parsees in spotless white, Jews and Arabs in dark rich silks; Klings in Turkey red and white; Bombay merchants in great white turbans, full trousers, and draperies, all white, with crimson silk girdles; Malays in red *sarongs*; Sikhs in pure white Madras muslin, their great height rendered nearly colossal by the classic arrangement of their draperies; and Chinamen of all classes, from the coolie in his blue or brown cotton, to the wealthy merchant in his frothy silk crêpe and rich brocade, make up an irresistibly fascinating medley. . . .

The Kling men are very fine-looking, lithe and active, and, as they clothe but little, their forms are seen to great advantage. The women are, I think, beautiful – not so much in face as in form and carriage. I am never weary of watching and admiring their inimitable grace of movement. Their faces are oval, their foreheads low, their eyes dark and liquid, their noses shapely, but disfigured by the universal adoption of jewelled nose-rings; their lips full, but not thick or coarse; their heads small, and exquisitely set on long, slender throats; their ears small, but much dragged out of shape by the wearing of two or three hoop-earrings in each; and their glossy, wavy, black hair, which grows classically low on the forehead, is gathered into a Grecian knot at the back. Their clothing, or rather drapery, is a mystery, for it covers and drapes perfectly, yet has no *make*, far less *fit*, and leaves every graceful movement unimpeded. It seems to consist of ten wide yards of soft white muslin or soft red material, so ingeniously dis-

119

posed as to drape the bust and lower limbs, and form a girdle at the same time. One shoulder and arm are usually left bare. The part which may be called a petticoat – though the word is a slur upon the graceful drapery – is short, and shows the finely-turned ankles, high insteps, and small feet. These women are tall, and straight as arrows; their limbs are long and rounded; their appearance is timid, one might almost say modest, and their walk is the poetry of movement. A tall, graceful Kling woman, draped as I have described, gliding along the pavement, her statuesque figure the perfection of graceful ease, a dark pitcher on her head, just touched by the beautiful hand, showing the finely moulded arm, is a beautiful object, classical in form, exquisite in movement, and artistic in colouring, a creation of the tropic sun. What thinks she, I wonder, if she thinks at all, of the pale European, paler for want of exercise and engrossing occupation, who steps out of her carriage in front of her, an ungraceful heap of *poufs* and frills, tottering painfully on high heels, in tight boots, her figure distorted into the shape of a Japanese sake bottle, every movement a struggle or a jerk, the clothing utterly unsuited to this or any climate, impeding motion, and affecting health, comfort, and beauty alike? . . .

It is only the European part of Singapore which is dull and sleepy looking. No life and movement congregate round the shops. The merchants, hidden away behind jalousies in their offices, or dashing down the streets in covered buggies, make but a poor show. Their houses are mostly pale, roomy, detached bungalows, almost altogether hidden by the bountiful vegetation of the climate. In these their wives, growing paler every week, lead half-expiring lives, kept alive by the efforts of ubiquitous "punkah-wallahs;" writing for the mail, the one active occupation. At a given hour they emerge, and drive in given directions, specially round the esplanade, where for two hours at a time a double row of handsome and showy equipages moves continuously in opposite directions. The number of carriages and the style of dress of their occupants are surprising, and yet people say that large fortunes are not made now-a-days in Singapore! Besides the daily drive, the ladies, the officers, and any men who may be described as of "no occupation," divert themselves with kettle-drums, dances, lawn tennis, and various other devices for killing time, and this with the mercury at 80°! Just now the Maharajah of Johore, sovereign of a small state on the nearest part of the mainland, a man much petted and decorated by the British Government for unswerving fidelity to British interests, has a house here, and his receptions and dinner parties vary the monotonous round of gaieties.

The native streets monopolise the picturesqueness of Singapore with their bizarre crowds, but more interesting still are the bazaars or continuous rows of open shops which create for themselves a perpetual twilight by hanging tatties or other screens outside the side walks, forming long shady alleys, in which crowds of buyers and sellers chaffer over their goods, the Chinese shopkeepers asking a little more than they mean to take, and the Klings always asking double. The bustle and noise of this quarter are considerable, and the vociferation mingles with the ringing of bells and the rapid beating of drums and tom-toms, an intensely heathenish sound. And heathenish this great city is. Chinese joss-houses, Hindu temples, and Mohammedan mosques almost jostle each other, and the indescribable clamour of the temples and the din of the joss-houses are faintly pierced by the shrill cry from the minarets calling the faithful to prayer, and proclaiming the divine unity and the mission of Mahomet in one breath.

How I wish I could convey an idea, however faint, of this huge, mingled, coloured, busy, Oriental population; of the old Kling and Chinese bazaars; of the itinerant sellers of seaweed jelly, water, vegetables, soup, fruit, and cooked fish, whose unintelligible street cries are heard above the din of the crowds of coolies, boatmen, and gharriemen waiting for hire; of the far-stretching suburbs of Malay and Chinese cottages; of the sheet of water, by no means clean, round which hundreds of Bengalis are to be seen at all hours of daylight unmercifully beating on great stones the delicate laces, gauzy silks, and elaborate flouncings of the European ladies; of the ceaseless rush and hum of industry, and of the resistless, overpowering, astonishing Chinese element, which is gradually turning Singapore into a Chinese city! I must conclude abruptly, or lose the mail.

ISABELLA L. BIRD
The Golden Chersonese (1883)

121

1882

Coloured Lanterns and Singing Girls

*The Prince of Wales's two young sons, Prince Albert Victor and
Prince George (later King George V), set out to see the world as
naval cadets on board H.M.S. Bacchante, eventually reaching
Singapore the day after Prince Albert's eighteenth birthday. The
account of their voyage was compiled from their journals, letters and
notebooks at the Prince of Wales's request.*

Jan. 10th. – ... At 4 P.M. we landed at Johnstone's Pier, where Sir
Frederick Weld, K.C.M.G., the governor of the Straits Settlements
met us with Captain Tunnard, aide-de-camp, and Mr. George Browne,
private secretary, and where Mr. W.H. Read, the oldest inhabitant
of the colony, read an address on behalf of the European, the
Armenian, Arab, Chinese, Jewish, and Malay communities.

One address only was presented by all the various races to typify
the unity which pervaded the whole community. ...

The pier was covered in with greenery and flags, and there was a
great crowd of people. We drove off up to Government House,
crossing the river by the iron Cavenagh suspension bridge covered
with white and red drapery, and along the esplanade more than a
quarter of a mile long by the sea shore. ... Mangrove trees with
their skeleton roots fringe the shore, and betel palms, bananas, and
other tropic trees grow by the road side. Government House is outside the town at the top of a hill surrounded with beautiful gardens
and park; an imposing building, palatial in style and dimensions. On
the second floor is a fine large reception room with a deep marble-
floored arcade running for shade along on the outside. There are
punkahs working the whole length of the immense room, keeping it
beautifully cool. The broad staircase leading up to this is decorated
with a profusion of flowers and ferns, and everything seems cool
and airy. Many of the servants in the house are Chinese; but there are

besides Bengalee servants with white tunics and scarlet and gold-laced belts, and with broad, flat, scarlet hats somewhat like a cardinal's. . . .

Dinner was at 7.30 P.M., to which came the Siamese princes, the Maharajah, Captain Durrant, several members of the council – over thirty-eight guests in all. Afterwards we drove out through the Chinese quarter in Singapore to see the illuminations: coloured lanterns were hung all about, and the streets were inclosed under awnings so that no chance shower might interfere with the festivities. Across the streets were suspended illuminated fishes and birds and animals, both real and fabulous, very similar to what we had seen at Hong-Kong. In some places there were Punch and Judy shows where the puppets were shown behind ground glass, on to which thus only black shadows were cast: further on were stages with Chinese singing girls on some, and exhibitions of fighting men on others. We heard that the Chinese had spent over four thousand pounds in these decorations and illuminations. . . . We got home soon after eleven.

Jan. 11th. – Woke in the cool of the early morning to the sound of birds singing just like the chirping of sparrows at home. Somewhere down below, outside, the hours are struck on a gong with a clear and yet far-off sound. Breakfast at 7.30 A.M. and start at 8 A.M. to shoot deer and wild boar: though we ought to have started three hours earlier. Sir Frederick drove us in his own drag with a team of four horses. Mr. Osborne joined us from the *Bacchante* and Captain Durrant from the *Cleopatra*. It was very hot, the thermometer showing between 120° and 130° in the sun when we got down at Bukit Timah police rest-house, half-way across the island. We all trudged into the jungle on the east side of the road, and after going some little distance were posted singly along the hillside. In the first beat Captain Durrant got one boar and George saw one deer, who passed very close to where we were stationed, but with the exception of these no living thing stirred the stillness of the air. We sat for an hour in the partial shade; overhead the heavy clouds threatened rain. . . .

Jan. 12th. – Up early, but did not breakfast till 10 A.M. It is very hot this morning, and we quite realise that we are only about eighty miles off the line. Went into the town in a gharry; they are queer little carriages, and just hold two people sitting *vis-à-vis*. They are tolerably cool, as they have a second roof raised about three inches off the body of the carriage so as to allow of plenty of ventilation; the top is coloured white. The variety of oriental costumes, the quaint Chinese house decorations, their joss shrines, the shops, the

Mohammedan mosques, the Indian temples, the Malay fishers' houses on posts, and the general bustle and life of the streets, are all interesting and picturesque. In Commercial Square found a shop full of Japanese and Chinese *curios* and some lovely birds of paradise skins all bright yellow, from New Guinea. They asked over a guinea apiece for them; which is dearer than usual. . . . Going home we had a look into the native Malay town, the thatched huts in which are built on bamboo piles and staging over the water, just like the pictures of the lake-dwellings in Switzerland during the prehistoric times. There were lots of sampans with mats and awnings, fishing gear, shells, and fish, and many long black-haired, brown-skinned Malay men and children paddling and poking about.

After dinner there was a fancy dress ball, to which the people began to come at nine. The Chinese came in state apparel. The Siamese princes also were in full uniform, a sort of loose-fitting tunic, one mass of gold embroidery but not stiff like our lace, for the thread is worked in very fine and therefore yields readily to every motion of the body: loose cloth knickerbockers with white silk stockings complete the dress. The Maharajah and the Bandahara were both there resplendent in jewels. The fancy costumes of many Europeans were very cool and pretty. All the grounds round Government House and all the roads approaching it up the hillside were illuminated with strings of paper lanterns festooned from pole to pole, over 4,000 in number. All the façade of Government House was lit up, with rows of gas jets on the upper tier, but on the second tier with numbers of large painted Chinese lanterns, hanging in the verandahs and corridors. We climbed up right on to the summit of the house, and looked down on all the long rows of festooned lanterns radiating from it in all directions through the grounds, and afterwards went down among the trees and admired the many effects produced by the countless paper lanterns, of every shape and size, hung about in the larger trees up among the branches; the whole was as pretty as anything we have ever seen. The dresses were all very good. We danced every dance except four, and went to bed at 2 A.M.

PRINCE ALBERT VICTOR
&
PRINCE GEORGE OF WALES
The Cruise of Her Majesty's Ship
"Bacchante" 1879–1882
(1886)

1882

A Dutch Wife

A barrister by profession, Hugh Wilkinson was travelling with a group on board an ocean-going yacht, enjoying a five-month voyage round the world. Here is part of a letter dated Feb. 7, 1882 which he wrote home from the Hotel de l'Europe, Singapore.

De Bosco is at present trying to kill the mosquitoes, which have got inside his curtains round his bed; he says there are so many inside, that it would be far less trouble to "shut them in" and sleep on the sofa! They seem to make straight for the curtains, in which they either discover or eat a little hole, through which they then swarm, and, taking up their various positions inside, cheerfully and patiently wait for their victim. The temperature in the room is now (11 p.m.) only 82°, but it is a moist heat which makes it unpleasant. There are several lizards on the walls of the room: they are harmless little creatures to everything but flies and other insects, which they stalk and pounce upon in the most wonderful way. Last night we had a deluge of rain, and to-day two tremendous tropical showers; it rains here without exception nearly every day, and it is nearly the same climate and temperature the whole year round, and days and nights are of equal length. It is very steamy and hot, making one feel flabby and limp, and not giving one's clothes a chance of drying day or night. Some Frenchman somewhere says, that this tropical heat is so great that clothes of any sort are insupportable. "I make von bundle of dem, upon which I seat myself, and in a short time they are wringing wet." In the hotels about these melting regions, what is called a "Dutch wife" is always provided for one's nightly comfort. Don't be alarmed, it isn't what you are thinking of. My bedfellow and I very soon quarrelled, and, after a short but stormy acquaintance, I remained sole partner of the bed. A "Dutch wife" is an elongated bolster which one places between one's two ankles and one's wrists for as much coolness as is possible;

125

but if mine had been alive she couldn't have been more worrying. She seemed to be most awfully in the way, and as I could get no peace with her in bed, and as she was rapidly getting me out of it, I thought it better to bring matters to a crisis by a tussle and stand-up fight, which was ended in my favour by a vigorous kick, which sent her bang through the mosquito-curtains to the other side of the room. This was my first, and will be my last, experience of a Dutch wife. The same thing went on in the other room to the war-cry of "Bachelorhood or death." Talking of Dutch wives reminds me that we haven't had any butter since we left Europe. We would give almost the price of a king's ransom for some good brown bread and Devonshire butter. We had once or twice in India butter made from buffalo milk, but didn't care much for it; we could easily do without it, and after the first trial did so. The stuff on the *Ceylon* is like half-melted train oil.

For vegetation, winter and summer are the same; when the leaves think they have been on long enough they fall off; and when fruit takes it into its head to appear and ripen, it does so. . . .

Yesterday we inspected the markets, which were very interesting, the fish-market especially so, with all its quaint and many-coloured fish. There were the usual very large prawns, eight or ten inches long, and a thin misshapen-fish which looked for all the world like the tin fish at a pantomime at home; another fish, just like an old maid we have in our county, and quite as good-looking in the face; you have seen the fish in the Aquaria at home, nearly round, and about the size and shape of a football. We also saw many cuttle-fish, and little fish like whitebait; immense cockles, some very repulsive-looking king crabs, and some small black ones; a quantity of sea-snails of a most brilliant red colour, and very lively. Nothing new to us in the fruit-market. We are told that neither the mangosteen nor durian are yet ripe; of course we are very much distressed at this, but we have oranges, bananas and pine-apples to console ourselves with. Amongst the vegetables there are many we have never seen before, but recognise a great many, including lettuces, onions, tomatoes, sweet potatoes, and the bright scarlet chillies. The oranges all about these regions never change the colour of their skins, which are the same bright green colour, even when perfectly ripe.

The Chinamen, who are far superior to the other brown races here, are quietly elbowing them out of everything; they seem to be ubiquitous. It is so strange to see them at their grub, with their little basins close to their mouths in one hand, and their chopsticks, which they so daintily and cleverly use, in the other. All the servants in the hotel are Chinamen, and half a dozen of them have come into our rooms this morning on the pretence of doing one thing or another. They are all cast in the same mould, and are consequently exactly alike. We are only able to tell it isn't the same fellow by the slight diversity in his dress, and knowing that the same person would not be such a fool as to keep coming in half a dozen times to do what he might have done at once. The Chinaman is spoken of as being the best of servants, and is always addressed "boy."

We went to a Malay theatre in the evening, but it was so stupid and incomprehensible to us that we went to another one, a Hindu theatre, which was quite as bad, everything being to us so absolutely without any meaning, that they appeared to be a pack of lunatics. . . .

This afternoon we leave for Johore, the Maharajah having most kindly invited the passengers to a banquet, and afterwards to a ball, and to spend the following day there before leaving for Manila.

HUGH WILKINSON
Sunny Lands and Seas (1883)

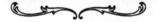

1886
Monkeys and Green Lizards

Otto Ziegele came out to Singapore at the age of twenty-two to be an assistant at the merchant firm of Brinkmann & Company. From the day he arrived he kept a diary.

June 1: Arrived in Singapore at 11.30 a.m., entrance to harbour splendid, all trees and small islands. Was fetched by a gentleman from the office, drove to office and then to the Hotel de l'Europe, where I met Forbes and family. Drove about with them, saw botanical gardens and said goodbye to Forbes family, who left at 10.30 p.m. for steamer. Therm. 85 with nice breeze going.

June 2: Got up at 6 a.m. My Chinese boy came and arranged everything, but owing to my not being able to speak Malay, I could not tell him anything.

June 3: Got up at 5 a.m., had a bath, not very nice as simply a beastly old tub. It rained pretty well all day long, fearful mess in the town.

June 4: Met a Mr. Bean of Liverpool, a nice fellow in same position as myself, at Syme & Co., only he for five years. Went home and then with Bean to rowing boat house. After dinner drove about in a rickshaw and went to bed 10.30 p.m.

June 5: . . . beastly hot and sweating like the very dickens, went at one o'clock with Mr. Specht to his house about 3 miles out of town, to the German Club. Rather a nice place, only they drink too much for me.

June 6: Went to Cathedral at 11 a.m. service, nice with communion but not many people present. Lunch at 1 p.m.; after lunch we drove to the botanical gardens with the intention of seeing and killing some snakes. Went into the jungle but did not see any, saw some monkeys and green lizards. Heat immense in sun, bought a few fresh cocoanuts,

128

which were very good. Went home and to evening service at 5½ p.m. Very nice singing, but a collection again (10 cts.).

June 10: After business, Bean and myself dressed and drove to Government House to see Lady Weld. We met a lot of people there, were introduced, had a drink and after a look about went home. Bean bought a small monkey for 2 dollars, a very amusing chap. Rain fell in the morning.

June 11: The Governor, Sir Fred Weld returned in the morning. After business called with Bean on Col. Dunlop, Inspector General of Police, who lives a long way out of town. Nice people, got back at 7 p.m., had dinner and then some music. Bean sings fairly well, piano bad.

June 12: Lot of rain in the morning, in business little to do, got home 1.30 p.m., had lunch and then went with Bean in a sampan to a cocoanut plantation, Tanjong Katton point. Had a long walk there, could have had as many cocoanuts as we like. We ate one and returned at 6 p.m. After dinner I went with Mr. Pellereau to the Union Hotel, heard some good music. Turned in at 10.30 p.m.

June 14: Got up at 6 a.m. and started at 7 a.m. well stocked with provisions in a large Malay sailing boat for one of the neighbouring islands. We had a glorious sail, landed at a very pretty place and had a good breakfast. We then had some difficult walking amongst high grass and low shrubs. Rowed to a holy island where we saw some Malay and Chinese praying churches. We had a grand bath, keeping pretty close inshore and started for an island with Sing. hospital on it, where we had lunch. We strolled about, killed a snake, 3½ feet long, coming down a tree, found some cuttlefish and shells and rowed home. We were rather tired and soon turned in.

June 18: After business went with Bean on board the steamer Espana. Had dinner with the captain, smoked actually 2 cigars and got home at 9 p.m.

June 25: Bean and I went at 9 p.m. to the ball of the German Club, but as far as dancing was concerned, not knowing any ladies, we did not get on well. The ball was very good but, of course, cuffs, collars and shirt fronts went to pot in no time, clothes simply got soaked. Had a rattling good supper, champagne ad lib and very fine. We left at 2 a.m. with 3 dances and the extras left to be danced.

June 26: Awfully fagged, got up at 7 a.m. Later heard that the fellows had stayed drinking till 6½ a.m.

July 3: Mahomeddan New Year's day, not a thing to do in business. I got away at 12 o'clock. In the afternoon we looked on at the continuation of the sports of the Eurasians, which were partly good; pole jumping 8 ft. 9 ins. easy; throwing cricket ball 95 yards. Some of the natives and hindoos were very funny and gaudy in their Sunday costumes, with bright yellow jackets, red and white striped trousers and faces painted blue (the cheeks).

July 4: Had an awfully heavy rain fall. Went to church as usual twice, afterwards we went to Boustead's young people's bungalow. Had a good dinner and some music on a Broadwood grand.

July 8: At 4.30 p.m. the Maharajah of Johore landed in front of the office. He had a grand reception with music and an address from the Chamber of Commerce.

July 9: Plenty of office work, enough to make anybody sick. Bean went to the ball of the Tanglin Club. I had a long walk and half a bottle of fiz. Bean's monkey was poisoned.

July 10: . . . at 5 rowed out in a sailing pair to see the boat races, which were very fair. At 7 o'clock we went to Boustead's young people, had dinner and then a game of penny nap, at which I won $3.80 (12/8). We finished the evening with some music.

July 11: Sunday. Had arranged to go for a bath at 5.30 a.m., but as Boustead's fellows never turned up, we could not go.

July 14: Awfully busy with mail, got away at 5.30. Went with Specht to his place and had a good game of tennis. We then went to the German Club and had a rattling game of nine pins till 1 a.m.

July 15: After dinner I went with some other chaps at 8 p.m. on board a small steamer for a trip to the lighthouse and back. It was a splendid moonlight night, we had a band on board and it turned out a nice trip. Got home at 12 p.m. very tired and sleepy.

July 16: After business played piano till dinner time. At 8 p.m. I went with an Englishman and two Dutch man-of-war officers to the botanical gardens to hear the concert by moonlight. It was a splendid night and we enjoyed it immensely till 11 p.m. We then drove to the Hotel de Louvre and heard some music. After every piece the girls come down and sit among the gentlemen, ready to drink any amount of beer, etc. We stayed till 12.30 . . .

July 17: . . . went with Bean up to Boustead's, where we had a good game of tennis. After that a stunning dinner and a game of cards till 1 a.m. We then had some music, a dance and some athletic sports, so that Bean and I only got home at 2.30 a.m. We were awfully tired.

July 23: Went to a small island on the left of the town, where they build ships. Bean wanted to buy a small boat. Stinks, etc., were immense; we soon went home.

July 24: Sailed to Tanjong Reu as the day before. Bean bought a Chinese sailing boat (sampan) for $14 without sails. We had a long talk with the English engineers on the island.

July 30: Got some orders for Damar from London and tried to get hold of some lots, only as soon as they see you want it they stick it on ever so much.

July 31: Very little to do; looked on at a cricket match between the club and the officers from Fort Canning.

Aug. 3: I had a little gymnastics with a German fellow and a good read.

Aug. 4: Footprints of a large tiger were seen four miles from the club.

Aug. 5: At 5 p.m. Bean and I went to Tanjong Rhoo to see Bean's boat, which is nearly finished. Stinks there are incredible, with pigs and rats all over the place.

Aug. 7: We received letters by first German mail steamer Oder, great excitement and grand tiffin on board.

Aug. 9: Bean and I went at 5 p.m. to Tanjong Rhoo, got Bean's boat launched and brought her over to the rowing club house, and in a pouring rain.

Aug. 12: I with some other chaps put the shot and the hammer. It was very jolly. We finished up with parallel bars.

Aug. 13: Great Chinese fete this evening, very amusing. They cover a table with all sorts of eatables, to their ideas the best of the best; they then lay knives and forks and pour out some brandy in glasses and put three or four chairs ready, in which their gods are supposed to sit and feed. Next to the chairs they put a basin of water and a towel, for the gods to dry their hands. Just near this they kick up an immense row with all sorts of infernal instruments and sing. Everywhere lanterns and thin smoking sticks, also incense (sandalwood etc.) is burnt. This is kept up all night and in Malay is called *Makan Besar* (large eating). The whole affair is very absurd, the gods seem to be very fond of liquor as each god has a large bottle of gin and three bottles of whisky or rum in front of him.

Aug. 16: The prices for board and lodging were put up from $50 to $60 a month, in consequence of exchange being so bad ($1 = 3/-½).

Aug. 17: I bought a Sergels piano for $300 . . . draft on the gov.

131

At 9 p.m. we had a meeting to form the start of an artillery volunteer corps, but owing to the poor attendance nothing definite was arranged.

Aug. 20: At 5 p.m. we had a meeting for the artillery volunteer corps, very poorly attended.

Aug. 22: Had a good look over the hotel to see if we could not find one room, where both of us might live in, to make it cheaper.

Aug. 23: Had a meeting of the artillery corps. We went through some drilling.

Aug. 24: Drove at 7 a.m. to Mount Sophia to look at the boarding house, Bean likes it and thinks of going up on trial, the house is nicely situated and clean. At 5 p.m. played tennis with a young German on the esplanade.

Aug. 25: Had a long talk about moving into the country; undecided about it yet.

Aug. 26: Rain all day long in torrents many places swamped. In the evening Bean and myself drove up to Clifton House (off Sophia Road) and decided at last to take one large room between us thereby saving a considerable amount. In the evening, we went to the Opium and Spirit Farmer's Fete. It was grand, a tremendous long table covered with every imaginable kind of food. At one end three priests say prayers loud all night long and at the other end a lot of chairs are arranged for the ghosts with heaps of cognac. We also saw a grand Chinese theatre which is awfully slow, although the costumes are very fine.

Aug. 27: Nothing on except in the evening at 5.30 p.m. our drill which was very poor only four turning up.

Aug. 30: Tremendous excitement in business; Mr. Gildemeister arrived looks well. Bean and I went to our new residence, Clifton House, and took a few things up, as yet the room has only the most necessary in it.

Aug. 31: We moved all our things and had our first dinner here; it was very fair, had a fine goose for one thing.

OTTO ZIEGELE
Singapore Diary 1886–1890

1887

Greater Town

*Li Chung Chu travelled south from Shanghai to visit his old friend,
the first Chinese Consul to Singapore. He wrote a full account of
what he discovered during his month's stay. ("Nanyang" which
means South Seas and "Silat" which means Straits are used here as
alternative names for Singapore.)*

Whenever a ship enters Singapore, flags are hoisted on Fort Canning
Hill and another hill on the western side to inform all merchants of
its arrival. By looking at the design of the flags, one will be able to
know what country the ship belongs to, what kind of business it is
engaged in, what type of ship it is classified to be, and which country
it comes from. These two hills are therefore known as flag-hoisting
hills.

There are forts on both flag-hoisting hills. The one on Fort Canning
Hill fires a cannon at noon every day for the adjustment of time by
the inhabitants. On every Sunday it changes its firing time to 1 p.m.
Besides, it fires again at 5 o'clock early in the morning and at 7 o'clock
in the evening to signify day and night.

Whenever there is a fire and the report is made through telephone
to Fort Canning Hill, the fort on the hill immediately fires a cannon
and a rocket. A flag is hoisted if it happens during the day, and lamps
hung if at night. The number of cannons and the colour of rocket,
flag and lamp imply which area the fire occurs. One will know where
it happens by looking at them. The fire brigade will start out immediately
after hearing the sound of a cannon. There are stand pipes along
the way and it is quite convenient to sprinkle the fire. Therefore no
big fire has ever occurred.

There are only a few temples in Singapore. The buildings of clan
associations or guilds are not magnificent. On the other hand, churches
are found everywhere. There are Roman Catholic churches, Christian

churches and Arabian mosques. Some are big, some are small, some are lofty and some are shabby. They number more than 20.

As far as prosperity is concerned, no area in Singapore can compare with "Greater Town". All the foreign firms, banks, Post Office and customs office are found along the seaside there. Although there are also bazaars in "Lesser Town", they are set up by the natives to sell local products and various foodstuff. Not a single big market is found there. At the northern side of the country there are plenty of parks and trees. It is the most serene and secluded region in the whole island. There is a place known as Kereta Ayer in "Greater Town" where restaurants, theatres, and brothels are concentrated. It is the most populated area where filth and dirt are hidden. No place in Singapore can compare with it. Along the streets gas lamps are on throughout the night. In front of every shop, there is a divine lamp hung over the door. During the nights of the second day and the 16th day of every month of the Lunar calendar, the divine lamp is lighted till 9 p.m.

Along Kereta Ayer, brothels are as many and as close together as the teeth of a comb. It is said that the licensed prostitutes registered at the Chinese Protectorate number three thousand and several hundred. Apart from these, there are countless unlicensed prostitutes and actresses. They are all Cantonese who were either sold at a young age and sent to Nanyang or were born and brought up in Singapore.

Year after year, little girls from Hong Kong are shipped to Singapore and sold to the brothels in rapid succession. The Chinese Consul took pity on them, and together with the local Chinese gentry, raised the matter with the British Governor who promised to order the Chinese Protectorate to draft certain regulations for the protection of these girls and for the establishment of Po Leung Kuk (Home for the Protection of Women and Girls) facilitating them to make investigation any time. Since then, this ill-practice has somewhat subsided. . . .

Restaurants are not abundant in Singapore. There are only one or two Cantonese restaurants and European restaurants respectively. Most of the feasts are held in the gardens of private homes with both Chinese food and European food served. Wines offered at such feasts are whisky, champagne and other European liquor. Glutinous rice wine and other eastern Canton products are getting less here. Shaoshing wine is like nectar, not to be found anywhere.

Inns are also very few here, far fewer than in Hong Kong, Canton or Shanghai. Whenever a steamship arrives at the port, nobody goes aboard to receive the new arrivals. They have to hire small boats

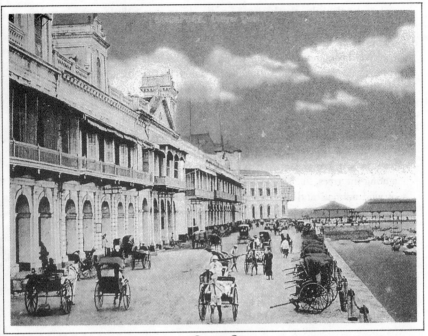

themselves in order to carry their luggage to the shore. Once they reach the shore they have in turn to get porters or horse-carts to do the same work. As most of the porters are Fukiens and the horsemen natives, the newcomers are unable to converse with them. They are quite easy to be swindled. It is, therefore, very inconvenient for a lone visitor to find accommodation here.

The price of opium in the South Seas is several times more than that in China. This is because the tax on it is heavy. In Silat, every mace of opium costs $2.00. It is said that in Java and Ache and other places, every mace costs only five dimes. However, the opium addicts are by no means rare in Silat. They are particularly abundant among the poor. For example a rickshaw puller can earn one dollar a day on average. After paying forty cents for hiring the rickshaw, there is still sixty cents left. If he is not an addict, he can lead quite a comfortable life. Unfortunately among ten rickshaw pullers there are hardly one or two who are not opium addicts. It is a great pity that they

135

toil so hard under the blazing sun merely to earn a little money, and yet this little money is entirely consumed by the chandu. . . .

The roads in the town are wide and even. They are repaired and restored throughout the year. Most of the bridges are made with fine iron. They look stronger than those found in the foreign settlements in Shanghai. The roads stretch in all directions greatly facilitating transportation in the town. Very often I go out for a drive at about 5 p.m. And when I travel from the seaside to the hill, what I see all the way are shady trees, fine grass and scattered flowers. Sometimes there appear in front of me a brook and a bridge or two or three huts, sometimes a storeyed building or a pavilion emerges obscurely among the trees. . . . Meanwhile the sun is about to set and the howling of wild animals and the crowing of roosters can distinctively be heard. I find myself as if among the mountains and streams in China, almost forgetting that I am in fact ten thousand *li* away from home.

LI CHUNG CHU
A Description of Singapore in 1887
(1895)
Trans. Chang Chin Chiang

1892

Carriage and Pair $5 Per Day

The Reverend G.M. Reith was Presbyterian Minister in Singapore from 1889 to 1896. He wrote regularly for the Singapore Free Press *and was a founder member of the Straits Philosophical Society in 1893, being its first Secretary and Treasurer. In his Handbook for visitors he recommends the following drive through town to the Botanic Gardens.*

There is more than one road to town from all the wharves, but the best is that skirting the shore, because of the cool breeze from the sea, and also because the road leads straight to the business part of the town. The syce must be instructed, if this route be chosen, to *Jalan tepi laut* (i.e. to drive by the sea shore). It is a well-kept road, laid with tramway lines, and the sea is kept in sight most of the way, a distance of three miles, from the P. & O. Wharf. It skirts a number of small laterite hills which are being fast quarried away for road-making purposes. Then Fort Palmer is passed on the right and the Chinese Quarter on the left, and the business part of the town is entered when Robinson Quay is reached. Collyer Quay is then entered, – an imposing terrace of offices with the convexity of the curve fronting the sea. At one end is the Teluk Ayer Fish Market, and at the other Johnston's Pier, whence communication is made by boat with the shipping in the Roadstead. The office of the Hongkong and Shanghai Banking Corporation is almost opposite the Pier. From Collyer Quay the passenger enters a triangular space at the junction of Collyer Quay, Battery Road and Flint Street, having on his right the Singapore Club and the Exchange (in one building), the General Post Office and the Shipping Office, behind which is the new Volunteer Drill Hall, and the remains of Fort Fullerton, the oldest of the town's defences. In the centre of this space is a large fountain presented to the Municipality by the late Mr. Tan Kim Seng, a wealthy Chinese citizen. To the left opens Battery Road leading to Raffles Square, in which are the offices of the other Banks . . .

Passing on, the visitor crosses the Singapore River by the Cavenagh Bridge to the Esplanade. To the left are the Government offices and Legislative Chamber, the Town Hall and Municipal offices (distinguished by a monument in front on the top of which is a bronze elephant, erected to commemorate the first visit of the King of Siam to Singapore), and the Supreme Court. Beyond these lies the Esplanade (*Padang Besar*) a large plain, encircled by a well-laid-out carriage drive. The Singapore Cricket Club, and the Singapore Recreation Club divide the plain between them for the purpose of cricket, tennis, bowls, and other athletic sports, and in the centre stands a fine statue of Sir T. Stamford Raffles, erected in 1887. A large part of the Esplanade occupies ground recently reclaimed from the sea; and it is now a favourite afternoon resort of the residents. On the landward side are the Hotel de l'Europe (*Punchaus Besar*) and the St. Andrew's Cathedral (*Greja Besar*). Beach Road goes eastward by the sea shore to the district of Kampong Glam, ending at the Rochore River, but the road now to be taken (Stamford Road) turns inland, and runs straight towards Fort Canning (*Bukit Bandera*), passing on the right, first the Raffles Institution, a school for boys, founded by Sir Stamford Raffles in the year 1823, and then the Church of the Good Shepherd (French Catholic); after which it turns northwards and from this point is called Orchard Road. The Raffles Library and Museum (*Tempat Kitab*) on the left, is first passed. It is well worth a visit, for the Library is one of the largest and most comprehensive in the East, and the Museum, which is being daily enriched by zoological, mineralogical, ethnological and archaeological collections from the Peninsula and the Archipelago, promises to be, in time, one of the finest exhibitions of its kind in Asia. The Reading Room and Museum are open to the public daily (Sundays excepted) from 10 a.m. to 6 p.m. There is a valuable collection of Oriental literature, called the Logan Library, access to which may be obtained by special permission from the Secretary.

Almost opposite the Museum is the Ladies Lawn Tennis Club (*Padang Kechil*), a prettily laid out garden where tennis is played from 4.30 p.m. till dusk. On the other side of the road is the Presbyterian Church (*Greja Kechil*) built in 1878, and a little farther on the same side, is a small Hindoo temple, used chiefly by the Dhobies (or washermen) who live in the neighbourhood, and who may be seen at work at any time of the day. Two hundred yards further on the Jewish Cemetery is to be seen, on the left, opposite Lambert Bros.' Carriage Works and Livery Stables. The gate of the approach to Government House is then passed on the right, beyond which is Koek's Bazaar, a row of native shops on both sides of the road. Between the hours of six and eight in the morning, this market presents a lively scene, hundreds of Chinese cooks and Asiatic women of many various nationalities come at that hour to make their purchases for the day.

Beyond the Bazaar, Orchard Road becomes a straight, well-shaded drive, leading to the European residences in the Tanglin district. On the left, almost hidden by the trees is a very large Chinese Burial Ground used by the Teo Chews i.e. Chinese hailing from Swatow; the visitor may perhaps overtake a funeral on its way thither, with the customary accompaniments of gongs to startle, and the scattering of gold and silver paper to appease, the demons which are supposed to be on the watch for the spirit of the deceased. Orchard Road ends at the entrance to the Military Barracks in Tanglin: and turning to the right into Napier Road, the visitor soon finds himself at the gate of the Botanical Gardens (*Kebun Bungah*).

These gardens were opened in the year 1873, and they are kept up by the Straits Government. Many varieties of tropical trees and flowers are to be seen there. In one of the ponds, a magnificent specimen of the *Victoria Regia* spreads its broad leaves over the water. There is a large variety of orchids and tropical ferns in the orchid houses; and close to these is the nucleus of a zoological collection of birds, snakes, and a few wild animals.

The charge for a carriage and pair is $5 per day, for a carriage with one horse is $3 per day; there being an extra charge in both cases, if the carriage is used after 7 p.m. . . . .

Hackney Carriages may be hired at the following rates (2nd class carriages):–

	$	c.
For any distance not exceeding half-a-mile	0	15
For any distance, exceeding half-a-mile but not exceeding a mile	0	20
For every additional mile or part of a mile	0	10

The fare for jinrickshas is 3 cents per half-mile for one passenger for a distance not exceeding 5 miles. At night (9 p.m. to 5 a.m.) an extra cent per half-mile may be charged. A jinricksha may be hired

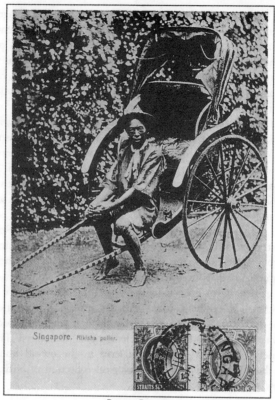

Singapore. Rikisha puller.

RIKISHA PULLER

for one day (i.e. not more than 8 hours, and covering a distance of not more than 10 miles) for the maximum charge of 80 cents, including charges for detention. An extra charge of half the fare is made when there are two passengers.

Visitors to Singapore are warned against the extortionate charges made by the gharry-syces. The above tables give the legal fares. When a dispute arises, the order to drive to the Police Station (*Pergi ka rumah pasong*) will bring the syce to reason, if his charges are exorbitant.

REV. G.M. REITH
Handbook to Singapore (1892)

140

c. 1896

These Rikisha Occasions

Minnie Farlow produced a series of articles, first published in the Singapore Free Press, which took a light-hearted look at Singapore life. Veiling her identity behind the initials M.F. and placing conflicting clues in different articles as to whether M.F. was actually male or female, married or single, she gained the freedom to observe as through the eyes of a newly-arrived visitor the ways of the resident expatriates which she gently satirised.

It was late one night; the horses had been out quite enough in the day, and something had "cropped up" that necessitated my hostess and myself going at once to a neighbour's house about three miles away, if the term neighbour is elastic enough here to apply to that distance. And we, by the bye, being already about the same distance from town ourselves, it was suggested that if we walked a short way we should easily find rikishas; and it was also suggested by my hostess, who is of a nervous disposition, that being a lonely part and a "dreadfully dark night," we should take the two terriers belonging to the household. Which we accordingly did, and started off. But the rikishas seemed to have done the same, for we had covered quite a mile before we came across one. There evidently was no chance of a second, so in we both got; and when the driver, or bearer, or whatever that particular sort of coolie is called – at any rate, I know he was a most miserable specimen of his kind – well, when he went off with us, I immediately felt that I ought to apologise for every pound of my weight. In fact, each stone of that "too, too solid flesh" (and yet I am not particularly portly!) seemed to lie like a stone itself on my conscience (it didn't on my hostess's though: she has been out too long!), as I surveyed the skin and bone that represented arms in our bearer.

It was his legs that concerned him most, however. Our wretched

141

canine followers declined to follow at all. They were aristocratic dogs, and having been accustomed to accompany their mistress in her drives, sitting in state in the vehicle itself, they could not understand being left outside. Or they may have laboured under the delusion that the rikisha man was carrying us off against our wills. But whatever the reason was, they made him so nervous with their darts at, and feints of attacking, his ankles, that we expected every moment to be dropped like the proverbial "red hot penny." On each side they went on with their growling and disapprobation until, in sheer pity for the man – a sort of "cruel only to be kind," when one thinks of the added weight – we had to take them in. From which point of vantage each dog surveyed him for the rest of the journey with doubts plainly expressed in one keenly-alert ear, and suspicion in the other! For my own part, I felt, when I alighted, that never had a rikisha man mopped himself so ostentatiously before, and that what *he* meant to express was simply volumes!

My pity for those men, when first I came, extended to what I then rashly imagined must be the monotony of their lives; but I soon found out that they have the daily – I don't think I should be far out if I said hourly – excitement of seeing how nearly they can manage being run over without that fact being quite accomplished. What language is used by the drivers of the carriages, as they pull their horses up on their haunches to avert the continually nearly-happening catastrophe, or what is said by the occupants of the rikishas themselves at these times, I am thankful that my limited knowledge of Eastern languages does not allow me to know. Suffice it to say that, when being driven home by my genial host himself, his involuntary observations, on these rikisha occasions (notably when crossing North-bridge Road) have been so far removed from geniality that I have had to request him to kindly make them in the Malay tongue!

M.F.
*Singapore Skits (in prose & verse):
a Visitor's View* (1896)

1898

First Glimpse of Barbarism

Delight Sweetser was a young American girl travelling round the world with her parents. They were fortunate to arrive in Singapore when the annual Hindu festival of Thaipusam was being celebrated.

Even the bad sailors made the journey from Hong-Kong to Singapore without quiver or qualm. But such January weather! I suppose we shouldn't look for frost in the neighborhood of the equator, but I haven't a Spartan spirit, and I like to grumble about the heat. We sat on deck all day with awnings to shelter us from the burning tropical sun while drops of perspiration trickled down behind our ears and along our spinal columns. We tried to get in the path of the faint, hot breeze and lay in our steamer chairs watching the glassy water lazily dimpling instead of rippling – too lifeless to do anything but breathe. Down in the dining salon the punkahs made the air endurable, but the cabins were stifling. In the evenings the moon was so fine that there was rarely any of the evening left and sometimes some of the morning gone before we could make up our minds to go to bed. The punkah is a sort of long fan hung above the tables, and swung by a servant, which is much used in the East.

The native of Singapore considers a bit of drapery, a brilliant turban and a silver ring around his ankle, and it may be his toe, ample costume for a hot climate. Perhaps he's right. . . .

The Chetties are interesting figures of Singapore streets. They come from India and are a rich and influential caste of money-lenders. There was a time when their word was as good as their bond, and in case of a failure the obligations of one were met by the others, but in the last few years some losses have been too heavy for them and they have lost the prestige they had. They are tall, dark, powerful fellows, scantily clothed in white. They shave their heads and around their necks they wear a massive ornament of pure gold. On their foreheads

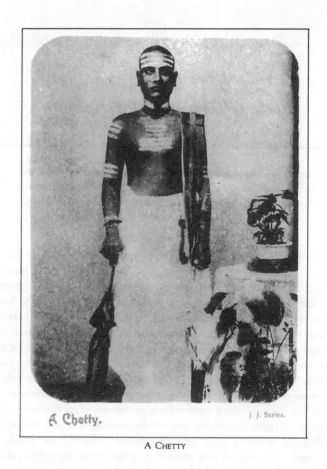

A Chetty.

J. J. Series.

A CHETTY

between their eyes they put a sticky substance which dries in a hard, round white wafer. I'm always thinking what capital ghosts they would make on a dark night, with only wafer, teeth, eyeballs and winding sheet in evidence.

It was our good fortune to see a procession which takes place annually when the god of silver is taken out for an airing and worshiped with many barbaric rites. We drove in a gharry from the hotel to the native part of the city where there is a Hindoo temple. The streets were full of picturesque figures in gay-hued clothes, bent on merry-making, apparently, more than worship, as holiday crowds are apt to be. We thought the Indian women with their lips and noses and ears pierced with silver and gold ornaments the most interesting. There were not many of them and the crowd was made up principally of men and children. Very few women are seen in the streets of Singapore, for the people have the Oriental idea of secluding them. I am speaking of the Oriental population, of course. There is a large English population, and some parts of the city are as English as England. . . .

At the end of the street where we entered we could see a gorgeous tinsel arch that seemed to be resting on the shoulders of a man, but he was so closely surrounded by the crowd that we could not get near enough to see him. If we stopped for a moment they crowded around us, and knowing that both cholera and small-pox were prevalent in Singapore, we didn't care to rub elbows with them. The man was evidently dancing, for the arch swayed and spun around and there was a jingling of bells. Afterward in the temple we saw a procession of dancers carrying the same gaudy arches and whirling in their frenzied dance. It was our first glimpse of barbarism, a revolting picture at which we gazed spell-bound. The men were bare to the waist and their mouths and noses and ears were thrust through with long silver pins which were wet with blood. Their arms and chests and backs were literally full of shorter silver pins which had been thrust so deep into the skin that they stuck and hung there like a bristling coat of mail. The men were staggering and half fainting from exhaustion and some were supported by a couple of attendants who prevented them from falling as they tottered on in frenzied gyrations. The worshipers in the tawdry temple gazed at them unconcernedly. Our gharry man brought us some of the sticky, whitish paste so that we might put a wafer on our foreheads. It was decidedly gray with dirt and we rather reluctantly adorned ourselves to oblige him. He didn't know enough English to explain the significance of it, but I afterward learned that the Hindoo decorates himself with the paste after his daily devotional ablutions and the style of adornment indicates his caste.

DELIGHT SWEETSER
One Way Round the World (1898)

1900

Pukkah Tuans

Many of James Rennie's recollections of the old days were first written as articles for the local newspaper; later he compiled them into a book. Here he recalls what it was like in Singapore at the turn of the century when he came out from England as a junior accountant aged twenty-five.

Yes, it seems a long time ago, does it not, and many rickshas have passed over Cavanagh Bridge since first I met you, Sunny Singapore....

General residential conditions have altered very much, there were no flats in those days; we of the "sinkeh" class, as the new arrivals were termed, lived in messes, very few of which are still in evidence, and happy days were spent in them. The Hongkong and Chartered Bank's juniors messed on the Bank premises, the former on the first floor of the previously existing building on the same site as now, and the latter in the building now vacant at the corner of Flint Street...

We juniors wore white duck tutup suits at $36 the dozen, white canvas boots at $2 the pair, we came to office in a rickshaw for the first few years and then sported a buggy and "waler," purchased from Daddy Abrams for say $250 complete with fly whisk and all, and a nice smart Sais standing on a dash board at the rear....

Tiffin was the "cold" from previous evening's dinner and was taken to office in a tiffin-box and consumed behind a screen in the office, no forty winks in a long chair afterwards then, but back to work until five o'clock.

There were no motors, trams, busses, or trains, and a journey to Serangoon for croc shooting or to Johore for a flutter at the gambling farm, was done by rickshas in relay, the fare being 3 cents a half-mile. If you want to hear something spicy about your forbears, give a rickshaw coolie 3 cents for a half-mile now, and he will astonish you with details of your ancestry if you understand the Chinese language.

146

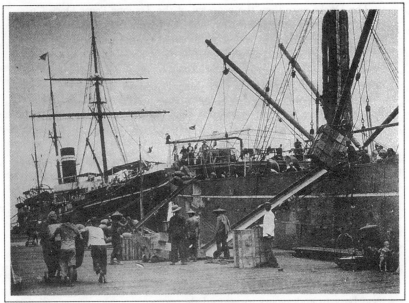

A great deal of riding was done in the early morning and Gallop Road was so named because it was there that we let the nag have its head for a decent gallop on turf.

The city streets are much the same except that Robinson Road and Cecil Street were hardly built upon, and Anderson Bridge not then built. The more urban roads are immeasurably improved and extended. Orchard Road had very few buildings beyond the present railway bridge, and Tanglin was largely comprised of stately bungalows with an average compound of 5 to 10 acres. Cairn Hill road was little more than an "estate" road leading to the Chartered Bank house, Dr. Galloway's, and the Lloyds.

The life blood of the Colony then, as now, had as its main artery, shipping, and though quite well catered for in those days, the amenities have since been very greatly improved.

The "Roads" in 1900 and until 1906/8 were open to the South West Monsoon, thus discharging and loading with Tongkangs was, at times, a precarious business, the dangers of which have been overcome by the Moles now in evidence.

147

The Docks were then the property of the Tanjong Pagar Dock Co., Ltd., which was expropriated by Government in 1904 and paid for in 1906 after arbitration in which many world experts were engaged. . . .

To many of the old timers including the Chinese it is still regretted that James Sellars' scheme for a navigable canal for Tongkangs has not been constructed from Kim Seng Bridge to the Empire Dock. The river, generally, appears to have been woefully neglected which might not have been the case had it been Batavia, Sourabaya, London or Liverpool; it would have been straightened, deepened, revetted, and given a back entrance to the Docks.

The Swimming Club was little more than an attap shed, no pagar, and Baddeley used to swim once a year from the Club to Johnston's Pier. The Cricket Club was, comparatively, a tin pot building and 90 per cent bar where pukkah Tuans Besar used to congregate. We had annual sports in those days, including cycle races and did not spend all our evenings bunny-hugging at hotels. The Gap was not known, though Lover's Lane in the Gardens, on a band night, had its devotees.

Girls of the genus white were few and far between and for about a week prior to the monthly dance at the Tanglin Club the telephone was busy in endeavours to secure lady partners.

The Germans gave us great times at the Teutonia Club, now Goodwood Hall, with Dances, Smoking Concerts, and Bowls, and once a year a delightful evening with a real Fair, very well got up, and "all the fun of the Fair," even to the biergartens.

We had no electric light and the use of gas was mainly confined to street lighting; in bungalow and office, kerosene lamps were used; no electric fans but something far more comforting by way of the punkah. Bananas were cheap and well ripened and the table always sported a dish of these, largely used to keep the punkah wallah awake on the verandah. We had no Cold Storage and no Sunkist Oranges but did quite well on ayam, Calcutta kambing, and local fruits Mangosteens, Chekoes, Dukoes, Pisang Mas, and Nanas.

We paid our boys $10 to $12 a month and cookie $15; a case of whisky cost $14 duty paid. Municipal Assessment was 8 per cent, rental values were one half of recent years rents, the Cricket Club was $1 per month, and stamp duty on a Conveyance 60 cts. per cent, so now you know what progress costs.

J.S.M. RENNIE
Musings of JSMR Mostly Malayan (1933)

1900–01

Flying Pigtails Everywhere

---

*While on a world tour, C.D. MacKellar visited Singapore, arriving at
the end of December and staying over the New Year period. Like so
many travellers, MacKellar was a guest at the Raffles Hotel.*

Singapore ways were new to me, though those who have dwelt in
the East will scorn my ignorance. My bedroom opened on the long,
wide balcony, and the space in front, partly enclosed and furnished
with table and chairs, was my sitting-room. The little swing-door of
the bedroom reached neither floor nor ceiling, so that it concealed
little of the room. There were two dressing-rooms and one of these
was my bathroom. It also had a little swing-door opening into the
inner hall. Chinese "boys," as they are called, passed to and fro, in
and out, regardless of me or my state of apparel. They paid no attention to anything I said, nor could I bar them out anyway. When I
wanted them I had to go and call them, and it so happened that I
wanted many things, for I was discarding all my garments worn on
the voyage, so that no New Guinea fever microbes should abide with
me, and what did on the ship would not do in smart Singapore. After
many appeals to passing servants, a languid Englishman in the next
balcony compartment said to me, "Excuse me, but these are my boys
you are ordering about." I apologised and asked how I could possibly
know that, as they seemed to use my room as a passage. He said they
were incorrigible that way, and explained that here one engaged at
once one's own Chinese boys to wait on one – they were not hotel
servants at all! He sent for an hotel servant for me for the meanwhile.

But now I am getting into the way of things here. I could not get
on without attention, so said to the hotel people I must have boys
to wait on me, and to "put them in the bill." Now I appear to have
six. They all look the same and I no longer lack attention or attendance.
I live a life of mingled laziness and overpowering energy, half in my

149

chair here and half tearing about Singapore in "rickshaws." My neighbour next door I do not see unless I advance to the front of the balcony. He then takes.his cigar out of his mouth and says "Ah!" He is always in his chair in exactly the same attitude with apparently the same cigar at the same stage. He never smiles and seldom speaks. Once as I was leaving the hotel my conscience pricked me and I thought perhaps he was ill and needed sympathy, so I returned the length of the huge building and along the balcony.

"Are you ill – are you well – are you all right?" I asked.

He looked astonished, then said, "All right."

"That's all right," I said, and departed, feeling satisfied and quite unable to prolong this interesting conversation. I have since discovered his vocabulary is limited to "Ah!" "Yes and No," "Pretty well," "Not bad," and "All right." It simplifies life.

A suspicion has just dawned on me that two of my attendants are his – they seem familiar somehow. But I don't know where any of them come from – if they are hotel servants, or his, or mine, or whose. I just accept the situation – it suits the climate. Anyway, already they are by way of "taking care of me," and grinning faces – all the same – and flying pigtails are everywhere.

My programme is, after my morning tub, to go and lie in my pyjamas with bare feet in my long chair. My tea is there, fruit, smoking material, books, and a Singapore newspaper. If I want anything I pull the nearest passing bell-rope – I mean pigtail – and point at something. They are wonderful, though; they know now even without my pointing. I notice, too, they have suddenly coiled their pigtails in an elegant coronet round their heads. I wonder why? I never see any one attending to my neighbour next door, but I can't help that. All my baggage is unpacked, strewn about, and in process of repair and cleaning. They did it all unasked, so I don't worry.

The first night I got into a rickshaw, and said I must be driven – or whatever you say in a rickshaw – very quickly all round the town. We tore along, scattering every one right and left; went first through a crowded street, and I had visions of painted ladies rising in balconies and rows of Japanese girls calling out in chorus, but we tore past unheeding and raced all over the place. "Here – hi!" I cried at last; "not so fast – stop!" whereupon my coolies came to a dead stop and nearly threw me out. I admire much the fat, rich-looking Chinese driving about in grand carriages with liveried Malay servants on the box, and I saw three stout Chinamen packed into one rickshaw, and

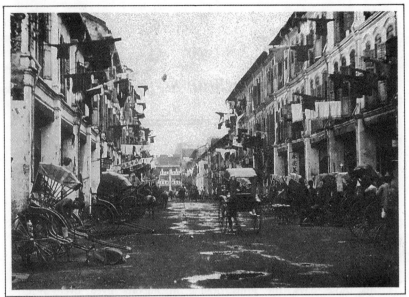

JINRIKSHA STATION

their coolie nearly fainting with the weight. These Chinese become rich and prosperous under our Government, but if they went to China would lose their wealth and their heads – but it will not be always so.

C.D. MACKELLAR
Scented Isles and Coral Gardens (1912)

Rickshaw Strike

At the age of twenty-three, Edwin Brown came to Singapore to join the merchant firm of Brinkmann & Company as their new assistant. It proved to be an eventful year.

My first days in the business life of Singapore were attended by drama. The first work that was given me was to take stock. It was a job that evidently was thoroughly disliked, and had obviously been left over for my arrival!

In those days, the firms dealing in imports lived over their "godowns." Collyer Quay was one long stretch of offices on the first floor (the only floor) of the buildings – the ground floor was taken up by the stores.

Having taken stock in a Manchester warehouse, I thought I knew all about the game and prepared to do it in my own way – a way obviously different, as the sequel will show, from what the staff was accustomed to.

I spent a perspiring day in the dirt and dark – for in those stores there was very little daylight and certainly no artificial light – and at the end of the day brought the result up to the office, quite proud of myself, only to be informed that I was forty bales of grey supers out in my reckoning.

The manager of the Import Department obviously did not think much of his new assistant, and I was sent down to take stock again. Another perspiring dirty day, with eyes open to make no mistake this time, but alas, the result was the same. The matter was now looked upon as serious, and I was haled before the Tuan Besar, who gave me a wigging, a lecture on carelessness, and a threat that if I didn't get proper results next time I might have to be sent home as incompetent! And so, with my tail between my legs, I made fresh arrangements to take stock.

On arriving at the godown early next day, ready to get down to it, I was greeted by an excited crowd of coolies and assistant storekeepers, jabbering to me in Malay (which I didn't understand). But I soon found out the reason, for there, on the floor of his office, lay the old storekeeper, dead! He had arrived before me, and hearing that I was to take stock again, and realising that the game was up, had taken poison and killed himself.

So I had been right after all; the forty bales of grey supers were in the books all right, but they weren't in the store! How long the swindle had been going on I never found out, or have forgotten, if I did know, but I have always wondered *how* the assistants took stock in the days before I arrived! I suspect they took a good deal for granted!

On the Wednesday morning we knew that the Queen, our great Victoria, was dead!

I can remember even now, and shall never forget, the arrival of that news. It was as if the heart of the great British Empire had stopped beating. Something had happened that seemed to be beyond the power of human intelligence to grasp. Men looked at each other and said nothing, but the expression on all faces was the same. "What is going to happen? To us? To the Empire? How can the world go on?" One had got so used to the fact that Queen Victoria ruled. No one out here could remember any other ruler, people had got to think of her as something fixed and unalterable, a necessity without which the Empire could not live.

The feelings at home at this sad time have been beautifully portrayed by Noel Coward in his great masterpiece, *Cavalcade*. It is not for me to attempt to add to that wonderful epic, but merely to try and show that the feelings that moved London at that time were moving the people of Malaya, as they were moving the whole of the British Empire.

I think the greatest tribute that can be paid to the memory of that great Empress, and to the grief and sorrow that moved the world at that time, is to point to the fact that youngsters of the present day, seeing *Cavalcade* on the stage or film, simply do not understand that scene. It is beyond them. It is, in simple fact, beyond anyone who had not arrived at man's estate before it happened, and who experienced it personally in all its tragedy and solemnity.

On Saturday, February 4th, the Memorial Service for the great

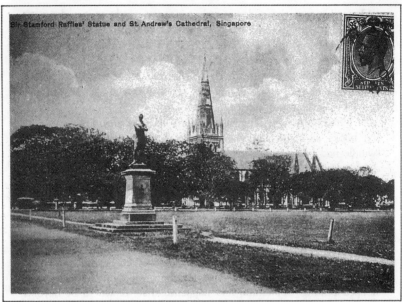

Sir Stamford Raffles' Statue and St. Andrew's Cathedral, Singapore

SIR STAMFORD RAFFLES' STATUE AND ST. ANDREW'S CATHEDRAL

Sovereign was held in St. Andrew's Cathedral. The time had been postponed until 6.15 p.m. to coincide with the time of the funeral at Windsor, and I suppose that never before had such an awe-inspiring service been held there, and possibly it has only been equalled once since, namely at the Armistice Service in November 1918.

It had been a dull, sunless day, making everyone conscious of the deep sense of awe and depression that was holding the Empire in bondage at the time, and the attendance at the service overflowed the Cathedral, filled the porches and a large portion of the roads round the building. . . .

It was calculated that, including those in the porches and in the grounds, from 1,400 to 1,500 people must have been present, and certainly, if that estimate was correct, there never has been such an attendance at any service up to the present day.

And I am in a position to know, for the next week I joined the choir and have been a member of that body ever since. I had been unable to get into the Cathedral for the service, and had to be content with a place in the crowd outside the West Porch. But I

154

shall never forget the reverence and the solemn attitude of that crowd, many of whom, from their position, could see nothing at all, and hear very little but the singing of the hymns.

An interesting sidelight on the reverence and respect in which all nationalities held the late Empress is shown by the following paragraph in the *Free Press* of the day:

> "The appearance of the town of Singapore was remarkable. . . . Those who went through the native parts of the city on Saturday saw a perfectly silent town, as far as business went. So literally were the orders of the heads of the various communities to stop business carried out, that bakers in many instances ceased to make bread, and the food shops were shut up. Even the rickshaw coolies and bullock-cart drivers refused at first to go on the streets, as they said it would be *salah*. . . . But for the crowds of people going quietly about the streets, it seemed like a city struck with the plague."

So much for the death and funeral of the great Queen. It is a period of my life that I shall never forget. I have seen monarchs come and monarchs go since that day, but the thrill and the solemnity of that time is still with me, and will, I expect, remain.

On October 21st of this year there occurred a rickshaw strike; in point of fact, the last one that was ever seriously to upset the even tenor of Singapore's transport problem, and it is, therefore, of more than ordinary interest, and worthy of being recounted in some detail.

The strike was well arranged, and was complete. With the exception of a few private rickshaws, there were none out on the streets at all. Residents in these days can hardly understand what this meant to the inhabitants of thirty years ago. I suppose that 75 per cent of the Europeans used rickshaws then to get back and forth to office, and, for the Eurasians and other portions of the populace they were almost the only means of transport. Private carriages and public gharries – the latter expensive – were the only other methods before the trams and buses came in.

The day the strike occurred was windy, with patches of rain. The mail was in that morning, and the offices had to be reached somehow and there was nothing to be done but to "hoof" it. So away went the male portion of the population, carrying Chinese umbrellas and the inevitable tiffin basket, hoping against hope that someone would pass in a horse vehicle and give them a lift.

Imagine it, you who roll easily to office to-day in your saloon cars, imagine your predecessors trudging along Orchard and Grange Roads, their white boots covered with the red mud of a wet laterite road – a mud which stained! – and send a little prayer of thanks to the Mr. Austin and Mr. Morris and their friends who have delivered you for ever from such experiences as we had then! Happy was the man who owned a bicycle on that day of the strike.

The origin of the strike seems to have been a demand from the police that the men who pulled rickshaws should know something of the rules of the road. The Governor had had occasion, a few months before, to report one who had run into his trap, nearly causing an accident, and when the police made their reasonable demand, it was immediately concluded by the ignorant men that the Governor was out for blood. Actually, the police were right, for when Mr. Hooper, the head of the jinricksha department, summoned a meeting of rickshaw Towkays, about one hundred and fifty turned up and only two had acquired copies of the rickshaw regulations, which, printed in Chinese, were at their disposal.

At the close of the meeting, so little had the idea of more order penetrated the brains of those foolish owners, that they went away and told the pullers that the police were going to fine them $5 a head, an obvious lie, and so the strike began, the rowdy element threatening to smash the rickshaws of the peaceable men if they didn't join in.

Unfortunately, the matter did not end with the mere strike, and numerous instances of people on bicycles being pelted with missiles, and pedestrians assaulted, were reported, so much so that the police officers were ordered to carry revolvers, and many of the other ranks were armed in some way or another.

The strike spread to the gharry-wallahs, who were frightened to go on the streets for fear of being attacked, and as the day wore on the situation worsened, and the word went round that the Europeans would be advised to arm themselves, too. John Little's and Robinson's were besieged with anxious purchasers of small arms, and that day I purchased my first – and last – revolver. Whether these instructions came from the authorities or not I do not know, but it is quite certain that we were not prevented from carrying the revolvers if we had them.

That night things got very dangerous. Two or three of us escorted some ladies from Zetland House to their home in River Valley

Road, with our loaded revolvers in our hands, and then made our way to the end of Coleman Street to have a look at the Esplanade, which was like Hyde Park on a Sunday afternoon, except that the moon was the only light available. Rather a weird scene, that big open space crowded with excited crowds of Chinese.

The principal roads were well guarded with armed police, and police reserves were standing by at various central spots, but the night wore away without any serious trouble.

The morning broke gloomy, and soon the rain came down in torrents, but the coolies absolutely refused to work, and so we had to trudge dismally to office again.

That day there were some ugly scenes, and in Chinatown the police had to make charges, and shots were fired in the air to frighten the crowds. Along Rochore Road and in the district round the rickshaw station, the strikers were active and considerable damage was done.

The Governor then took a very firm attitude and summoned the Towkays to attend at Government House. He explained to them that they were on British soil, and what they could do in China they could not practise here with impunity.

The actual happenings at that meeting are not known, the papers rather contradicting themselves when reporting it. But the "rumours" of it, whether actually true or not, were generally accepted at the time.

It was said that His Excellency kept the Towkays waiting at Government House for about an hour, sending in biscuits and drinks to them. When he did appear, he talked to them affably about the weather, etc., and said it was very nice of them to call and see him. After a short while he excused himself, saying that he was very busy, and just as he was leaving the room, turned to them and said: "Oh, by the by, gentlemen, there's a rickshaw strike on in town. There's also a boat leaving for China to-morrow. If that strike is not stopped before the ship leaves, you'll be on it! Good morning."

Whether this actually happened or not I cannot say, but certain it is that next day the strike was called off, and in a few hours the vehicles were out on the streets again, and Singapore quickly resumed its normal aspect.

EDWIN A. BROWN
Indiscreet Memories (1934)

157

1901

The Cleverest Monkey

*At the peak of a brilliant career, Sir Frank Swettenham was ap-
pointed High Commissioner for the Federated Malay States and
Governor of the Straits Colony. After years of dealing with Malay
royalty, Sir Frank found that some of his first duties as Governor
were to entertain British – and Russian – royalty visiting Singapore.*

It was the middle of February, 1901, when I reached Singapore and
took over the Government from my brother Alexander, who had
been Administrator since the lamented death of Sir Charles Mitchell.
I had been warned that T.R.H. the Duke and Duchess of Cornwall
and York would visit Singapore with a large party in H.M.S. *Ophir*,
and there was little enough time to make the necessary arrangements
for their reception and entertainment before they arrived in April.
Besides Their Royal Highnesses, and Captain Winsloe and officers of
the *Ophir*, there were nineteen members of the Royal party, which
included H.H. Prince Alexander of Teck, and it was impossible to
accommodate all of them in Government House. We made the
most of the space available, but had to arrange that about six of the
guests, and practically all their servants, were housed elsewhere; the
guests with members of the community, and the servants in hotels.
For such a memorable occasion the Rulers of the Federated Malay
States were invited to meet Their Royal Highnesses, and with their
ladies and numerous followers were lodged in furnished houses prepared for their accommodation. The Sultan of Pêrak brought his
mounted Sikh escort and his State carriage, and the latter – drawn
by four horses with English postilions – served to carry the Duke
and Duchess on arrival, departure, and other formal occasions. I
was given to understand that the travellers preferred rest to efforts
made with the best intentions for their entertainment. So beyond
the reception on landing at Johnston's Pier, where Their Royal

Highnesses were received with a Guard of Honour, a Salute, and the cordial welcome of all classes of the community, the only demonstrations were a large dinner party at Government House, and a Torchlight Procession organized by the Chinese to march through the grounds and past Government House from which the Royal Party had a close-up view of a remarkable display. . . .

There was one little incident which would have disappointed me had not the Duchess saved the situation. I wanted to show Her Royal Highness something distinctive of Malaya, so I sent to Malacca to secure the attendance of the cleverest coco-nut gathering monkey in that Settlement and of his owner. When they arrived, I arranged for a demonstration in a suitable grove of palms on a picturesque road, and drove the Duchess and her ladies to see the monkey do his turn. On the way I explained that the monkey would climb the tree and throw down any nut selected by the spectators. I had seen it done a hundred times without failure, but I must add that, on those occasions, what was always wanted was a young nut full of cool, delicious milk. When we reached the grove the monkey and his master were already there, only waiting for the order to open the proceedings. A palm was selected and the monkey – with a long cord round his waist and the slack in his master's hand – was told to climb. He did so with remarkable agility and when he reached the fronds and the nuts he looked down for orders. These were shouted to him and with a little string-pulling he was soon above the chosen nut with his hand upon it. Then the order was given to throw the nut down; but the monkey looked bewildered and began to move away, neither threats nor cajolery having the smallest effect on him. Another nut, rather higher up, was then picked out, and the monkey led to it by the same means with the same result. I felt like the conjurer whose trick has been a complete failure, and I was very annoyed with the owner of "the cleverest monkey nut-gatherer in Malacca." The monkey had now returned to earth and was sitting behind his master, who looked very glum. I said: "I asked for the best monkey in Malacca and he can do nothing. What was the use of bringing him here to show Her Royal Highness his skill?" To which the owner replied: "He *is* the cleverest monkey in Malacca; he can collect three hundred nuts in a day. But he is trained to collect ripe nuts, not green ones. All those selected were green and he knows better than to gather them."

When the position was explained to the Duchess, H.R.H. said she

159

thought it was much cleverer of the monkey to be able to discriminate between green and ripe nuts than just to twist off the chosen nut to which he was led by voice and by pulling the string. So everyone was happy and the monkey and his owner returned triumphant to Malacca, having upheld the honour of that ancient Settlement. . . .

Whilst I was absent in Penang, a Russian war vessel put into Singapore Roads. The Captain had recently died at sea, and the cruiser was under the command of H.I.H. the Grand Duke Cyril, who ranked as a Commander in the Russian Navy. My A.D.C., following the rules in such cases, called upon the Acting Captain and explained that I was away. When I returned to Singapore I expected that as the Grand Duke was on service he would call at Government House, but he did not do so. I told the Russian Consul that I wished to invite His Imperial Highness to stay at Government House if, in accordance with practice, he would call on me. Then the Russian Consul came to see me and said the Grand Duke wished to stay with me, but he thought that I should call on him first. I pointed out that His Imperial Highness had arrived as the acting captain of his vessel, and as such the rule about calling was quite definite, to which his Consul replied: "Yes, but after all, he is a Grand Duke." I said that sooner than make a difficulty over such a trifle I would pay the first call, which I did, and the Grand Duke returned it immediately, and then came to dinner. About the same time the Grand Duke Boris also visited Singapore, but as he was not on service there was no trouble. I took him to a famous green pigeon shoot, at an island off the East Coast of Johore, where the pigeons fly from mainland to island every evening between 5 and 6.30 p.m., and give capital sport to guns stationed in boats off the island. The pigeons pass the day on the mainland, where they feed on fruit they gather from jungle trees, and, according to Malays, the reason why they fly to the island to roost is because the island has no monkeys. The jungle has many, and they are said to catch the sleeping birds. I don't think the Grand Duke enjoyed the shooting party. He was wearing a new sun hat, and the steam launch which carried him belched drops of oil, mingled with the smoke from its funnel, and spattered the hat, so that his attention was divided between shooting pigeons overhead and attending to his hat.

SIR FRANK SWETTENHAM
Footprints in Malaya (1941)

1907

A Favourite Place for Europeans

To mark the new century, a series of descriptive books on the Empire was produced, and the one on British Malaya included a section giving the latest information for tourists in Singapore.

The visitor to Singapore will find no lack of objects of interest and beauty. One of the first sights that tourists generally make a point of viewing is the Botanical Gardens – among the loveliest institutions of the kind in the East. . . .

Another very beautiful spot which should certainly be visited is the Thompson Road reservoir, where a fine stretch of water is seen amid thickly wooded slopes. This is about four miles out of town. Again, there is the Gap – a delightful drive along a ridge of hills overlooking the sea that occupies about two hours.

As for other drives of interest, one can hardly go wrong in taking a hackney carriage for a couple of hours – it only costs the equivalent of 3s. – and leaving it to the sweet will of the driver to carry you whither he lists; for the roads of Singapore, whether along the sea-fringe or running into the interior of the island, are so good, level, and beautiful as regards their arboreal dressing, that it does not matter very much in what direction one turns. . . .

In the city proper the visitor will find innumerable sights and scenes to attract his attention and retain his interest – the street life alone possessing a wonderful variety of colour and picturesqueness. The hub of the town in a commercial sense is Raffles Place, sometimes called Commercial Square. This has been the business centre of the colony ever since it was founded. Here at one time were situated all the big shipping and trading houses, banks, and stores. Nowadays it cannot suffice to accommodate more than a mere fraction of these establishments, and they have consequently spread to the neighbouring streets and to Collyer Quay, which is now almost wholly

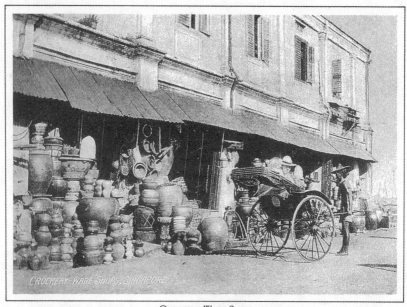

CROCKERY WARE SHOPS

occupied by the shipping firms. The Square itself still remains the great shopping rendezvous for the European section of the community, and is a very busy place from nine o'clock in the morning till five o'clock in the afternoon, after which hour, however, it is almost as deserted as the Sahara. In the day-time, the never-ceasing stream of traffic – carriages, gharries, rickshas, and foot passengers, with their wealth of colour, quaintness, and movement – makes a wonderfully interesting kaleidoscopic procession. High Street, which is only a few minutes distant, is the home of native jewellers and silk-sellers, and should not be missed by the tourist in search of curios. Crossing High Street at right angles is North Bridge Road, which with its continuation, South Bridge Road, forms the longest thoroughfare in town and the main artery for traffic. Along its entire length, this street is lined with Chinese shops of all conceivable kinds – silversmiths', ivory workers', rice shops, pork shops, eating houses, hotels, and what not – whilst the side streets leading from it are simply thronged with stalls on which a medley of foodstuffs and pedlars' wares are exhibited. In North Bridge Road is situated a

Malay theatre where plays, ranging from "Ali Baba" to "Romeo and Juliet," with musical interludes, are nightly presented before crowded houses. This is a favourite place for Europeans to visit who want to see and hear something out of the common. The plays are presented in Singapore Malay, and, even though the visitor may not understand the dialect, he will have no difficulty in following the action of the pieces. There is also a Chinese theatre near at hand, where a seemingly interminable play goes on all night, and where it is amusing to observe the cool way in which the spectators will sometimes stroll across the stage right among the actors, to find some more convenient point of view or to exchange greetings with a friend.

In South Bridge Road and in Orchard Road, also, there are two Indian temples which are always open to inspection by the visitor. Small Chinese temples and joss-houses abound all over the neighbourhood, and the tourist will find a half-hour visit to any of these places interesting and instructive by reason of the many strange rites and sacrificial customs to be observed by the habitués. In the Chinese joss-houses one of the things that strike the European visitor as most curious is the way in which edible offerings are made to the "joss." A Chinese lady, resplendent in silks and jewellery, will come along, perhaps accompanied by her young sons and attended by a coolie bearing a huge basket replete with all sorts of delicacies, prominent among which are roasted ducks and coloured Chinese cakes. After the necessary formalities have been gone through, the edibles are duly placed out in festal array in front of the particular "joss" whom it is sought to propitiate. Then the worshipper burns some joss-sticks and coloured papers, after which the coolie sweeps all the good things back into the basket and the party go off rejoicing to feast upon them at home.

While entering the harbour, the visitor will doubtless have been struck by the numbers of small islands which lie around Singapore. Some of these are British, others are Dutch. For the most part they are uninhabited except for an occasional fisherman, but they are favourite places of resort for local hunters, who find there abundance of wild pig, pigeon, and quail; while the creeks are generally capable of affording sport to the "shikari" in quest of a crocodile. Should it happen that the steamer enter the harbour from the western end, the visitor will pass through a narrow channel between the island of Singapore and that of Pulo Brani, on which are situated the largest tin-smelting works in the world. On the Singapore

163

side of this channel is the commencement of the Tanjong Pagar Docks, the recent expropriation of which by the Government created quite a stir in shipping and commercial circles.

The tourist should make it part of his programme to pay a visit to Johore, the capital of an independent native State of the same name on the mainland opposite the island of Singapore. Here are situated the headquarters of the State Government and the Sultan's Palace, or Istana, as it is called – a luxuriously fitted residence, full of rich and valuable furniture, paintings, and furnishings, not the least valuable of which is the famous Ellenborough plate, acquired in England by the late Sultan. The main objects of attraction in Johore, otherwise, are the gambling-shops, which are daily and nightly crowded with Chinese – both men and women – engaged in play at the favourite games of "fan tan" or "po." These shops are licensed by the Government, to whom they are sources of enormous revenues. In Singapore no gambling is allowed – indeed, the anti-gambling laws are very strict – so that Johore is the rendezvous for all the "inveterates" from the neighbouring British settlement, with which it is connected by a railway and steamboat service, the whole journey between the two towns occupying a little over one hour.

Eds. ARNOLD WRIGHT & H.A. CARTWRIGHT
"Information for Tourists"
Twentieth Century Impressions of British Malaya (1908)

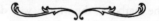

164

1908

In High Spirits

Count Fritz von Hochberg, a Prussian nobleman, enjoyed his second visit to Singapore while on a leisurely tour of the East to escape the Northern winter.

We landed at Singapore on Sunday, 16th February, at 1 P.M. I can't say how pleased I was. I love Singapore, it is a charming place. As we drove from the boat to the hotel I was astonished to see how much had been done to the place since I was there four years ago. Lots of these swampy, feverish places round the harbour and the Chinese quarter have been filled up and planted, and it made the place ever so much nicer looking. But it is a nice place altogether, and with its pretty cathedral on a large green lawn, under beautiful large trees, and its pretty, shady quays and avenues and fine Town Hall and other public buildings, looked most picturesque and pretty. . . .

February 18th. – We drove out to Buka Tima in a motor I had hired. The drive was lovely. First past all the pretty bungalows, then past the Botanical Garden, and then out into the jungle where all sorts of picturesque Malay or Chinese villages were nestled in the rich green vegetation, and large pineapple or rubber or cocoa-nut plantations. After one hour's drive we got out at the foot of Buka Tima Hill and walked up. It was beautiful high jungle, and the vegetation was really magnificent in its rich luxuriance. Marvellous high evergreen trees and creepers grew in graceful garlands from tree to tree, and underneath was a thick undergrowth of all sorts of bamboos and lovely ferns and mosses. Huge butterflies, as large as sparrows, flew and hovered over the thick ferns, but they were not as bright coloured as ours, they had more transparent wings as if they were made out of thin *crêpe*, and were mostly marked grey and white-spotted like a guinea-hen.

The road ascended in well engineered curves round the hill, and the top was reached in three-quarters of an hour's easy walking. How much weaker I must have been when I did it four years ago! Then I had the feeling that it was almost two hours' stiff walking, and now it is nothing.

At the top the bungalow was empty, and after calling to see if anybody was in, we quietly ascended the little staircase, up which I had followed the young couple who then lived in it four years ago, and we came out on the roof-terrace from where one has a lovely view over the whole island and all the surrounding islands and on to the mainland, where the white Mosque of Johore and the Sultan's palace are easily seen. While we were sitting admiring the lovely view, and remarking that the only thing was that it was a pity nobody was here to give us any refreshments, as we had got rather hot on the climb, an old Chinaman appeared on the roof and asked if we wanted anything. He was the caretaker. "Yes, of course!" – what had he got? "*Only* pineapple," he said quite apologetically; and of course we were delighted, and he soon brought us an enormous dish full of the juiciest, best pineapple I think I've ever eaten. It must have been at least three. We made a regular feast. . . .

Wednesday, 19th. – We drove in the same motor to Johore. The drive was lovely, first as far as Buka Tima of course the same, then magnificent jungle down to the sea, where we took a ferry-boat and were rowed across by a sulky Chinaman. It took about forty minutes to paddle across this arm. The heat was intense, and under a scorching sun we walked on the other side and into the Sultan's Park, past two sentries, who presented arms as we passed. I expect we had no right whatever to go in there, but as, to the trio's great amusement, I militarily thanked the sentries for their salute, bowing graciously to them and touching my hat with the two fingers of my left hand, they let us all quietly pass, and we found the walk in the shady and well laid-out grounds of his Highness the Sultan most pleasant, and enjoyed it thoroughly. Finally we ended at the Mosque, and, after taking off our boots, were admitted. It is most disappointing from inside, as there is really absolutely nothing to be seen. A huge, brand new, plain building, with white marble floor, and the walls and large columns holding the ceiling only whitewashed and painted like coloured marble; horrid, crude, stained glass windows. As we came out a terrific thunderstorm was coming up, and we hurried back to the shelter of the hotel. Some rikshahs came to meet us, and I put Mrs F. in one, and induced the Chinaman to let me have the shafts of her rikshah, and off I trotted with her. It was much easier than I thought. Fritch photographed us like that. We just arrived at the hotel when it commenced to pelt, and it pelted on the whole afternoon, as if it were never going to stop. So, after patiently waiting till almost six – we couldn't stop there the night, not having anything with us – we climbed into covered rikshahs and were driven in the pelting rain to the landing stage. There a funny thing lay in the water, entirely covered over with matting tied to a high pole. It was our boat! I shouted out, and the dripping matting began to move like a reptile, and at one end our sulky Chinaman appeared. Unnecessary to say that he was very cross by now, and no wonder, and our childish hilarity made him still crosser. So he paddled his boat up to the landing stage, and we crawled in on all fours under the matting. Inside the boat was perfectly dry, but it was rather narrow for us four, and very low. Of the Chinaman we only saw the feet and calves, as he was paddling standing up at the end where he had opened enough of the matting to let his body pass. Arrived at the other side the rain had stopped, but the tide having gone out, there we lay at least thirty yards off the shore and a dirty, muddy, slimy bit of water-mud between us and the dry land. Another Chinaman came wading out and offered to take us on his back and carry us across, of course the only thing to do. Mrs F. refused boldly, but finally was persuaded by her husband to let herself be carried across, after having made me promise her that I would not *photo* her. I kept my promise not to *photo* her, but could not resist the temptation to make a hurried sketch of her on a visiting-card, as I was left the last to be carried over. The sulky Chinaman saw it and shrieked with laughter. He laughed so heartily, I haven't for a long time seen anybody laugh like that. He tapped me on the back, he beat his hands, he held his sides, he simply doubled up with laughter, and couldn't caress and pat me enough. It was so funny, that I, already in very high spirits, couldn't help laughing too, and there we both were laughing like two madmen. Of course the other three already deposited must really have thought us mad. Once on the mainland, I showed my sketch, and they all began to laugh, because I must say, in its roughness and spontaneity it was very funny. Mrs F. didn't mind, but the old Chinaman, who hadn't stopped laughing, made us understand through unmistakable signs that he would not have anything paid for his boat hire, if only I would give him the sketch. Mr F. wanted to have it too, of course, so the only thing to do was to copy it out quickly, and as soon as we had given the Chinaman the original he went off laughing still, and never turning round for his fare, which of course I wanted to pay him. I shouted after him, and our chauffeur told it him in Chinese, but he only waved his hand as if to say, "never mind that," and splashed back through the mud into his boat, looking at the sketch and laughing all the time like a happy child. Surely never before has one of my works been so appreciated, nor ever will be again.

We arrived at the hotel at 8 o'clock, and it was pitch dark, and the roads were torrents. One drove in water.

The next day, 20th February, was lovely and sunny, and so, after shopping . . . we took the motor after lunch and drove out towards Beech View, but past it where the road branches off. It was a lovely drive past all sorts of plantations, mainly cocoa-nut palms, which really are magnificent, and then in a large Chinese village where an open theatre was going on. We stopped to see it. The actors were just painting their faces, and mostly seemed to represent devils or such, but it was really interesting to see how ingeniously they painted their faces with black, white and red water-colours, and really succeeded in making marvellous unrecognisable masks of their faces, otherwise harmless enough. Then they proceeded with their dressing, and some had lovely old-gold embroidered costumes, some huge coloured wings and dragons' tails, crowns, etc., etc. The acting and singing was more a contorted sort of devil's dance in which the real Devil displayed much power with funny high jumps. None of the audience, though, paid the slightest attention to the acting. We were the theatre to them, and they did not take one eye off us. Especially my having sketched the face of the man who I thought painted himself best, interested them greatly. . . .

We then ended at Beech View Hotel, where we had tea, and our child (Healy) played with the monkey. That evening after dinner we again went in rikshahs for a drive round the Main Quay, where all the smart Chinese and Malay society go for a cool evening drive, and an endless stream of carriages and motor-cars passed us filled with bejewelled and beflowered ladies, all in rich and brilliant silks and satins, all in native costumes, while the pig-tailed men walked on foot on the outside avenue. All that evening a really deafening pandemonium of firing of crackers had been carried on in front of some Chinese houses near the hotel. They went on for over an hour. It was to frighten the evil spirits away, as it was full moon, and

168

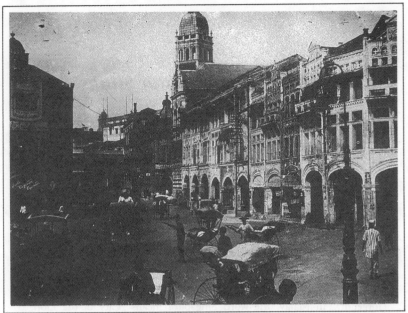

so the last day of the New Year's festivals. — And beautifully the moon had been coming up over the sea and the forest of masts of thousands of djunks lying there in the old harbour.

COUNT FRITZ VON HOCHBERG
An Eastern Voyage (1910)

1911–12

Chinks, Drinks and Stinks

After the boredom of serving in his father's store in Perth, Australia, young James Redfern set out on a series of hopeful quests for easy money, one of which led him to Singapore where he soon found himself in unusual employment.

Singapore – the melting-pot of the East! Whenever I had met white men I had heard tales of this strange polyglot city; the abode, some said, of Chinks, Drinks and Stinks; others, less cynical, told me: "You'll like it, or you'll hate it, but if you go there you'll never forget it." In Malay, the word Singapûra means "City of the Lion," but behind the British lion's back a good deal goes on which he knows nothing about, as I was soon to learn.

. . . I arrived there without very much money, knowing nobody and having not the slightest idea of what I should do, other than await the arrival of the balance of my cash from Batavia. My first steps were in the direction of a cheap hotel. From the wharf I took a rickshaw along Anson Road, through the business quarter and was eventually deposited at the door of Raffles Hotel. Two minutes' investigation assured me that I was *not* staying there. Thence I was taken to the Europe, an even more inviting and expensive caravanserai! Finally I managed to get the rickshaw boy to understand that this particular *tuan* was one of the lesser Lords of Creation who wished to rest at a cheap (and therefore despicable) hotel in possibly one of the less fashionable quarters of the city. Back we went, down to the maze of narrow streets by the harbour, streets hung with a myriad signs in Chinese characters, in curious English, in French even, the inner purport of which was not hard to guess. We stopped several times until at last, tired of hotel-hunting, I paid the boy off outside a rather dingy three-storey building bearing the superscription: "The Anchor Hotel." Proprietor: A. Ferenc.

I went in, interviewed Mr. Ferenc, who turned out to be a Hungarian Jew of enormous proportions, sloppily clad in *sarong* and pyjama jacket and always in a state of perspiration, and booked a room. In spite of the man's repulsive appearance there was a twinkle in his little pig-eyes which decided me. I heard later that he was quite a well-known figure in certain circles in Singapore at that time, but how he got there and who he really was I never discovered. Anyway, I installed myself in a reasonably clean room and set about the business of waiting for the Batavia mail and investigating the city's possibilities.

Up to that time it was the biggest place I had ever been in and my tours of exploration had plenty new to show me. Night life, especially in the vicinity of my hotel, was both varied and lurid, for we were within fifty yards of the notorious Malabar Street, the centre of Singapore's extensive "red-light" area.

The other "residents" in my hotel interested me considerably. There were two English seamen, whose ship was undergoing repairs in the harbour, a little Jap who went out every day at seven and returned at nine with the regularity of clockwork, and, best of all, an Australian! . . .

"You stay here, Jim," he said. "You'll pick up all the money you want in Singapore if you do what I tell you."

I decided to take his advice in the end. What I had already seen of Singapore fascinated and attracted me, and foolish as it may sound I started there and then to embark on a brief career of wasting my substance in riotous living. We went everywhere in the less reputable quarters, the gambling hells, the opium dens, the brothels in Malay Street, Japanese wrestling matches, the Chinese theatre, eating-houses, cock-fights, enjoying all the more sordid delights of the city. The Raffles and the European Club remained closed books to me, but I daresay I saw more of Singapore through Perce Wilmer than the planters and Government officials who had been in the city for ten years. It was at a cockfight that I met Mr. Lee Fong.

Wilmer and I had gone to witness this spectacle in a covered court-yard behind a certain Chinese restaurant not very far from The Anchor Hotel, he attending in a professional capacity – laying odds – while I was a privileged spectator. We were the only white men in an audience of perhaps seventy or eighty Chinese, all well-to-do business men from their appearance.

The cockpit was a biggish circle laid with matting and roped off rather in the manner of a boxing ring, complete with umpire. The

171

fancied birds were enclosed in bamboo cages and first of all passed back and forth among the spectators for examination. As the first match came on, the birds were held breast to breast by their owners until a signal from the umpire bade them loose their hold and the rival roosters went for each other like twin furies. I have never seen anything so exciting in my life and, considerations of cruelty apart, I still believe this is the most thrilling spectacle devised by man for his entertainment. The backers remained completely poker-faced and apparently unimpressed as feathers flew and the sharp steel spurs manoeuvred for the death-blow. Not a hint of emotion was on anyone's face, except mine!

The moment the match was done, however, a babel of noise ensued, the faces broke into smiles or scowls and the "bookies," including Perce Wilmer, paid out. We watched ten matches in all and I saw very considerable sums of money change hands. When it was all over, the proprietor of the pit handed round little cups of *hocshu* to everyone and the spectators dispersed. I noticed, however, that Wilmer was in deep converse with an enormously fat Chinaman, beautifully dressed in a long embroidered coat, and presently he called me over to him.

"Mr. Lee Fong has been inquiring about you, Jim," he said. "It seems that you're getting quite a reputation for high living already. He's a very successful business man and I took the liberty of mentioning you might be soon looking for a job," he added with a meaning wink. . . .

We went inside to the restaurant and spent the next hour talking of everything under the sun except a job. Just as we were leaving, however, Lee Fong said: "If you are in need of employment at any time, Mr. Ledfern, I should be velly pleased to have a talk with you at my office." . . .

My association with the firm of Lee Fong and the man himself was, to say the least of it, a most extraordinary one, and I suppose there are few white men who have had the opportunity of coming in such close contact with the life of the Chinese community as I did.

. . . Wilmer was right about this fat old Chinese. The style of "General Merchant" comprised countless activities on his part, ranging from money-lending, pawnbroking and banking to a flourishing import business and a private information bureau. I soon learnt that there was practically nothing that went on in Singapore among either the white or coloured population, but Lee Fong knew about it. He had his agents in practically every club, hotel, office and even houses in the city. Gossip and tittle-tattle picked up in every quarter of the city was brought to him by servants, clerks, compradors, rickshaw-pullers, and goodness knows who else, paid for if worth it, and discreetly filed away. Some time, he said, it might be useful. I don't wish to imply by this that he was a professional blackmailer. He was far too clever for that, although I don't think it would have interfered with his scruples. But there are other ways of turning information to good account sometimes, and I believe he was used by the police occasionally. He employed me to watch his money-lending interests, or more truthfully as a sort of genteel debt-collector. A lot of his business in that direction was done with the young men who came down from some God-forsaken up-country plantation and got themselves into financial trouble through having too good a time. They went to Lee Fong in preference to some street corner Parsee because he had built up his connection on straight dealing and not too exorbitant interest. Moreover, he was a substantial man, which encouraged confidence, and his discretion was unimpeachable. My job was the administration of polite reminders, and what he called inspection of security, which was nothing more than observing the subsequent activities of his "clients," and informing him if they appeared to be gambling too heavily, involving themselves with women, or otherwise endangering the prospects of the return of a loan! As a white man this was a great deal easier for me to do than for him; my presence in certain circumstances would pass unnoticed where his would attract attention and for obvious reasons my prestige as a *tuan* would give me accidental "contacts" no Chinese could ever make. For this I was given a generous expenses allowance and a far better salary than I could have got as a sub-assistant overseer on some rubber estate, which was about all I had hoped for.

I was amazed at some of the names on his books.

JAMES REDFERN
Looking for Luck (1930)

1915

Mutiny

When Indian troops at Singapore mutinied on February 15, security on the island became a problem. In London The Times reproduced the following letter from "the wife of an English official, who with her two infant children had to seek refuge in the old prison." The Times added: "The riot was caused by a portion of the 5th Light Infantry, who 'ran amok,' murdering Europeans. It was promptly quelled by the local forces, assisted by landing parties from British and Allied ships, though not without further loss of life. Some 30 Europeans, military and civilian, were killed."

Punishment Cells, The Gaol, Singapore.

... The above address may be a shock to you, but wait until you hear of our experiences! On Monday, 15th, S____ and I were having our tea, and I had just said that after all this is the safest place for me and the babies and I had better not go home until next year, when the telephone rang and Mr. H.'s voice, very agitated, told me to be on our guard as two soldiers from the Indian Regiment were "running amok" and shooting all Europeans. He had just seen the doctor from the hospital (the very nice man who operated on S____ and was so kind) shot dead in his car just below our house. We had heard shooting all the afternoon, but thought it only the Chinese New Year cracker firing, though some of the bullets had actually been whistling across our "park-like grounds." S____ then telephoned to the gaol and found things were much more serious than we thought, and that it was a mutiny of the Indian Regiment and the native gunners, the only regular troops left to defend us. All the German prisoners were said to have escaped, and names of friends whom we had been seeing only a few days ago were mentioned as killed or wounded.

Night was coming on and it would have been madness to stop in our isolated house, with the jungle so close round, so we went down to the gaol to see where the whole family could go for the night, and this room amongst the punishment cells seemed to be the safest place, except the old prison, which was already crowded with all the warders' families and wives and children of men at the docks. We took the babies and amahs and all the absolutely necessary impedimenta wanted down the hill in the pitch darkness, with a guard of three warders armed with loaded rifles, and felt and looked just like the cinema pictures of Belgian refugees. Our one room is generally used as a chapel for the Christian prisoners, and Christie and I slept behind the altar rails and the amahs on the wooden forms, while "Robert Francis" reposes (fitfully) in his "pram." Mrs D____ and another woman, wife of a police-inspector, have camp-beds; they came in late that night for shelter, too.

In the morning, just as one was beginning to forget the fears of the past night, the firing suddenly began again just outside the gaol, and the order was given for all women and children to go to the old prison. I was making the babies' food at the moment and dashed across with the boiling milk and any other indispensable article of infants' food and clothing I could carry . . . the amah had already run across with Christie. Such an awful scene of horrible dirt and squalor we found there: the building is old and not in use generally, except for executions – the floors thick with dust and the ceilings with cobwebs. Every room had families of poor, tired women and filthy, tired, howling, hungry children – one ghastly child of three, half-witted and having screaming fits and convulsions all the time, added to the general air of misery. We camped ourselves in a room where there was space to turn round – but the mutineers were firing at us from the hill opposite and we had to keep away from the window.

All day the volunteers and those officers of the regiment who had not already been murdered by their men were hunting the brutes down and the prisoners were brought in here, 99 altogether. In the evening the ringleader was caught and S____ and some of the officers kept him and a few of his pals in the courtyard just below our windows while they decided what to do with him. He is a native officer, an awful-looking beast with a fierce face and wuffy black beard. He had been wounded in the shoulder and his picturesque white draperies and turban were soaked with blood. The English officer says he is a very bad character and hopes he will be shot or hung. At present he is in a cell just below us and is spending his evening reciting the Koran in a monotonous sing-song voice.

175

Yesterday afternoon some of the women ventured out to their houses to get food, but were shot at and scuttled back again. I had just taken off some of my things in the hopes of getting cool and resting while the babies slept, but hastily dressed again for fear of having to make a sudden dash for the Old Prison again. A French cruiser had left here last week, and a marconigram was sent asking her to come back at once. She arrived to-day and the French sailors have done splendid work in rounding up the remaining mutineers, assisted by the Japanese Volunteers and the men from H.M.S. Cadmus. We hear there has been a little battle on the racecourse to-day and they have got all the rebels surrounded – so that soon we ought to be quite safe.

I couldn't stand the dirt of the same old clothes on any longer this evening. S____ was dying for a bath, too: so, armed with a rifle and with two warders both armed, we marched up to the house. Everything looked as usual, only a horrible garment soaked in blood just outside the garden to remind us of the dangerous time we have been through. Such a sweet, pretty young bride who was out at Changi with us the other day was killed with her husband. One of our warders died from his wounds yesterday, and 21 English men and women were buried yesterday afternoon. The Sepoys went quietly about in couples with haversacks full of ammunition and deliberately shot at every European man or woman they saw – we do not know how many are wounded yet. All the women and children are ordered on board a troopship, but S____ telephoned to Government House that we are safe here and I should hate to be sent off to that dreadful crowded ship away from S____ and not knowing what is happening on shore.

"The Singapore Riot"
The Times, March 26, 1915

1915–17

War Intermezzo

An architect and prominent member of the local Swiss community, H.R. Arbenz was six times president of the Swiss Club in Singapore and appointed Honorary Consul in 1929. Here he tells of his experiences during the Great War when the Swiss were suspected of pro-German sympathies.

When I arrived in Singapore in April 1915, the last of the 40 Indian mutineers were shot outside the prison, opposite the present mortuary, in accordance with the martial law then in force. It was a public execution meant to act as a deterrent. The whole hill, where the General Hospital now is, was full of spectators. I can well remember how 110 volunteers were called up to shoot the 22 men; it was on a beautiful Saturday afternoon. The Provost Marshal of the time was a volunteer officer, Major Thompson called the "Red Thompson," formerly a director of the Gas Works and subsequently a planter in Sumatra. Altogether 40 men were shot; one was hanged, because he had assassinated Lieutenant Montgomery by stabbing him with his bayonet when he was endeavouring to raise the alarm over the phone. A Mohammedan dealer of Indian nationality (who had a shop) in the Adelphi Hotel building was also hanged, because he had had the "brilliant" idea of writing to Constantinople with the request for the Turkish Navy to occupy Singapore. The mutineers belonged to the only regiment then present in Singapore. It was said that they were going to be sent to Gallipoli against which, as Mohammedans, they objected. The Germans at that time were interned in the Tanglin barracks and some of them took advantage of the opportunity and made use of the panic by escaping, amongst them Lauterbach, an officer of the "Emden". The Governor, Sir Arthur Young, publicly declared during a military parade on the Padang that the Germans had had nothing to do with the mutiny.

177

... the Swiss were decried as pro-German, with the result that a number of house searches were made, also at my place. One morning the Detective Station phoned and requested me to call there. A police officer received me, made me empty my pockets after he had held up a warrant to my face. With the exception of a photograph which he required for his album of criminals he kept nothing back. After that we had a rickshaw ride together to my room in Cavenagh Road. He was a comical fellow; one does not encounter anything quite as "schofeles" (mean, shabby) everyday. He accepted a whisky soda without much ado, then asked me for a cigarette which, as a non-smoker, I could not provide. After that he took his own cigarette case from his pocket without showing the least compunction. The procedure was repeated with the matches. He then "nosed" through my writing case, deciphered the blotting paper with a mirror, à la Sherlock Holmes. Finally, after he had seen my cheque book and rummaged through everything, I asked him what he was looking for, as I might be able to satisfy him. He then started to speak out freely. He had a copy of the Swiss Military Journal on him, on which my military rank and address was printed, a circumstance which he combined with the fact that I was the President of the Swiss Club and that he had heard of my conducting arms' drills at the Club. I was able to mollify him on that score, as the 12 members had no intention to surround Singapore and capture the place, seeing that we much preferred Jass (cards) to drills. He had furthermore "found out" that I had been engaged to go to Java for the purpose of building fortifications there. I replied that I would be most grateful to him if he could secure such a contract for me.

When he left empty-handed I mentioned that he would certainly hear from me again, to which he grinned and replied that martial law was prevailing and that I would be up against a brickwall. On the same day I went to see our Consul, but, oh weh! (woe betide!) he dared not undertake anything in the matter, as he claimed not being "persona grata" with the authorities himself. So I took my courage into both hands and called on General Rideout whom I happened to have met socially. I put the case before him and noticed immediately that this suited him down to the ground, as the Military and the Police were at loggerheads because of disputed competence. He immediately asked me who had signed the search warrant, but I had to admit that, while I had seen my name on the warrant, I had not seen the signature, the paper having been folded over. The General dismissed me with the request to call on him again in a few days at Fort Canning. The matter got clarified: there had been no signature on the warrant; the General only was authorised to sign. Sherlock Holmes was accordingly second best and had to leave the arena for good.

Another search took place after some Swiss were found to be talking in their Swiss dialect in the Hotel van Wijk. In every hotel someone of the Secret Service was stationed at that time. In the van Wijk it was Kotawalla of the Indian Civil Service who alleged that he knew the German language and that he had understood some of the words. Also one Levy frequented the hotel who claimed to be an American and tried to ingratiate himself with us and preferably spoke German. I always thought he was an informer.

Another "War Intermezzo" took place in 1917 when the Allied asked the Japanese to return the conquered Kiaochow (bay) and the Shantung province to China. As they refused to do so, the Chinese started boycotting Japanese goods and looted the shops, burning some of the loot in the streets. The Japanese fleet which at the time guarded Singapore harbour offered to suppress the rebellion, but the British authorities wisely declined and recalled the British gunboat "Cadmus". With a few machine guns the disturbances were quelled.

We also had the visit of the Tsarist fleet of Russia. Such a "Voellerei" (high living, gluttony) Singapore has not seen since. The Commander and the officers stayed at the Europe Hotel, drank champagne only and were full to the hilt. The Commander himself fell down the stairs and damaged his "facade." The sailors slept off their drunkeness anywhere. Some lay over the tram rails near the Meyer Mansion and stopped the traffic; others lay on the display cabinets of the shops in the Adelphi building, broke the glass and got injured. The local police did not have the courage to interfere.

The stay at hotels became more and more unpleasant for the Swiss so that the advantage of having a Club of our own increased steadily in importance. Every Sunday there was a curry tiffin at the Club. One was off to Bukit Tinggi already in the morning, some on foot, others on horseback via Thomson Road and along the reservoirs, yet others by rail from Tank Road or Newton station to the Holland Road Halt, near the bridge across the Bukit Timah canal. There were various accidents, once a salto mortale (somersault) of horse and rider into the reservoir, another time the horse had to be destroyed as it broke a leg in a swamp. As varied and as interesting the

179

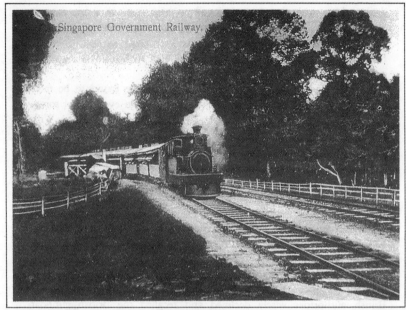

GOVERNMENT RAILWAY

ways to the Club proved to be, as unpleasant and uninteresting was the way home. One usually waited for the last train and rushed down the hill, and, if one was lucky, caught the train, but no seat. The Chinese had usually taken possession of the carriages and sprawled all over the first class compartments. They travelled on free tickets received from the gambling farm in Johore. Very often, however, the train left the moment one got to the foot of the hill, when there was nothing left but to straggle home on foot and benefit by the sobering effect of walking.

H.R. ARBENZ
A Personal Memoir
One Hundred Years of the Swiss Club
and the Swiss Community in Singapore 1871–1971
by Hans Schweizer-Iten (1981)

180

1920

A Real Man-Eater

The Great War stimulated a demand in the U.S. market for films showing far-away places. So, Alexander Powell together with a cameraman journeyed through Borneo, the Dutch East Indies, Siam and Indo-China filming exotic locations. While passing through Singapore he heard a traveller's tale well worth repeating.

The tiger is to Johore what the elephant is to Siam and the kangaroo to Australia – a sort of national trademark. Even the postage stamps bear an engraving of the striped monarch of the jungle. There is no place in the world, so far as I am aware, save only a zoo, of course, where one can get a shot at a tiger so quickly and with such minimum of effort. In this connection I heard a story at the Singapore Club, the truth of which is vouched for by those with whom I was having tiffin. Shortly before the war, it seems, an American business man who had amassed a fortune in the export business, and who was noted even in down-town New York as a hustler, was returning from a business trip to China. In the smoking-room of the homeward bound liner, over the highballs and cigars, he listened to the stories of an Englishman who had been hunting big game in Asia. The conversation eventually turned to tigers.

"Johore's the place for tigers," the Englishman remarked, pouring himself another peg of whiskey. "The beggars are as thick as foxes in Leicestershire. You're jolly well certain of bagging one the first day out."

"I've always wanted a tiger skin for my smoking room," commented the American. "Could buy one at a fur shop on the Avenue, of course, but I want one that I shot myself. Think I'll run over to Johore while we're at Singapore and get one."

"But I say, my dear fellow," expostulated the Briton, "you really can't do that, you know. We only stop at Singapore for half a day –

181

get in at daybreak and leave again at noon. You can't get a tiger in that time."

"There's no such thing as 'can't' in my business. Business methods will bring results in tiger shooting as quickly as in anything else," retorted the American, rising and heading for the wireless room.

A few hours later the American's representative in Singapore, a youngster who had himself been educated in the school of American business, received a wireless message from the head of his house. It read: "Arriving Singapore daybreak Thursday. Leaving noon same day. Wish to shoot tiger in Johore. Make arrangements."

Now the representative in Singapore knew perfectly well that his promotion, if not his job, depended upon his employer getting a tiger. And, as the steamer was due in four days, there was no time to spare. From the director of the Singapore zoo he purchased for considerably above the market price, a decrepit and somewhat moth-eaten tiger of advanced years, which he had transported across the straits to Johore, whence it was conveyed by bullock cart to a spot in the edge of the jungle, a dozen miles outside the town, where it was turned loose in an enclosure of wire and bamboo hastily constructed for the purpose.

When the steamer bearing the American magnate dropped anchor in the harbor, the local representative went aboard with the quarantine officer. Ten minutes later, thanks to arrangements made in advance, a launch was bearing him and his chief to the shore, where a motor car was waiting. It is barely a dozen miles from the wharf at Singapore to Woodlands, the ferry station opposite Johore, and the driver had orders to shatter the speed laws. A waiting launch streaked across the two miles of channel which separates the island from the mainland and drew up alongside the quay at Johore, where another car was waiting. The roads are excellent in the sultanate, and thirty minutes of fast driving brought the two Americans to the zareba, within which the tiger, guarded by natives, was peacefully breakfasting on a goat.

"He's a real man-eater," whispered the agent, handing his employer a loaded express rifle. "We only located him yesterday. Lured him with a goat, you know . . . the smell of blood attracts 'em. You'd better put a bullet in him before he sees us. One just behind the shoulder will do the business."

The magnate, trembling with excitement for the first time in his busy life, drew bead on the tawny stripe behind the tiger's shoulder. There

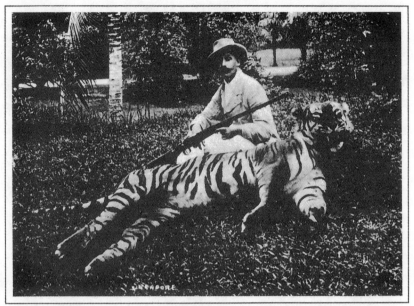

MAN-EATER

was a shattering roar, the great beast pawed convulsively at the air, then rolled on its side and lay motionless.

"Good work," the local man commented approvingly. "It's only an hour and forty minutes since we left the boat – a record for tiger shooting, I fancy. We'll be back at Raffles' for breakfast by nine o'clock and after that I'll show you round the city. Don't worry about the skin, Sir. The natives'll tend to the skinning and I'll have it on board before you sail."

Now – so the story goes – after dinner in the magnate's New York home he takes his guests into the smoking room for cigars and coffee. Spread before the fireplace is a great orange and black pelt, a trifle faded it is true, but indubitably the skin of a tiger.

"Yes," the host complacently in reply to his guests' admiring comments, "a real man eater. Shot him myself in the Johore jungle. Easy enough to get a tiger if you use American business methods."

E. ALEXANDER POWELL
Where the Strange Trails Go Down (1921)

183

1921

Globe-Trotters Killing Time

Under the headline "On the Empire Trail", The Times in London published an article "from the pen of a widely-travelled Special Correspondent who has recently returned to England from a visit to Malaya".

If I say that Penang did not disappoint me I must couple with it, I'm afraid, the remark that Singapore, which, for so many years, I had joined with it in imagination in one sunlit picture, did. It belied the promise of its name, and that, in a sense, is my only excuse for writing about a place already so much written about and so well known. I used to sit in Kuala Lumpur – midway between the two, half a day by rail and ferry from either island – and think to myself, "There's another and bigger Penang down there; it can wait a little." And yet my instinct was not quite at fault, for I did begin to have a sort of growing doubt before ever I saw it. It was an unformed doubt, but, in the uncreated words in which it arose, the image gradually altered. It became, somehow, more commonplace. I don't know whether it was the talk of others or whether the near-by presence of a town can impress its personality on the intuition. I rather think it can, but, however, that is of small importance before the fact that Singapore is not a Penang. It has neither the inward nor the outward colour. It is heavy with commercial zeal, it hangs upon the sea like a drab giant, greedy and overfed. To find the charm of Singapore – for it has a charm of its own – you must consider it from another angle.

It was a fine morning on which I approached that island. The ferry is only a matter of a few minutes over a mere two miles (they have already begun the construction of a causeway), and, once you are on the other side from Johore Bharu, there is still an hour's run in the train through hilly jungle, which offers no kind of hint of the great town ahead. Singapore lives on its shipping; it thrives, so to speak, upon the brine of its harbour, but pales before the massy forests. Yet it has its compensations; it looks forth daily upon the ships of the world, and with the steady eye of its fixed prosperity it gazes for ever upon the wandering populations of the sea. The bristling sight from the esplanade is indeed one to astonish an inhabitant of the interior, and the hotels of Singapore are eternally crowded with globe-trotters killing time with a distracted expression of haste. They have a quaint cosmopolitan flavour on one issuing from the seclusion of Malaya, and I could not help watching them attentively, as though they were just going to order taxis to take them to Charing Cross.

Singapore is now in the throes of its first real modern spell of trade depression, and it is rather pathetic to observe its slightly bewildered air of forced optimism. On the surface things appear much as usual; its hotels are still crowded, from the Europe, Raffles, and Van Wyck downwards, its 4,000 motor-cars are still busy, its streets are still seething, but beneath it all there is a creeping lassitude upon its activities. The shipping, though immense, is not what it was of old; the godowns are full of raw goods it does not pay to export and finished goods the up-country traders cannot accept. The town, like a camel in the desert, is living on its hump; is living on hope. Its huge fabric reminds one, unironically, of a whited sepulchre; it is the product of trade, and, without trade, it is a mere shell. Well, of course, not altogether, because its geographical position is its ultimate value; but to a large extent Singapore is in urgent need of the reviving breath of commercial enterprise.

It was curious how soon one became unconsciously aware of all these things, just as it was curious how, as I walked the streets of Singapore, I felt weighing upon me the vast islands of the Dutch East Indies, Borneo and Sumatra, that hem it in on either side and await, in turn, the development of their incalculable riches. The world needs more and more the produce of the tropics, and these half-virgin islands, small continents in themselves, will be playing their part when Singapore has sunk to trivial importance through the cutting of the Siamese Canal. I do not say that that will be to-morrow; I do not say that it will be in 20 years' time. But it will come. They have waited long, these islands; they can wait a little longer.

Of an evening the European population of Singapore gives itself over to exercise, while rich Chinamen roll through the famous gardens in their cars, and contemplative strangers bask along the sea front. As for the lowly native life, that goes on for ever unchanged,

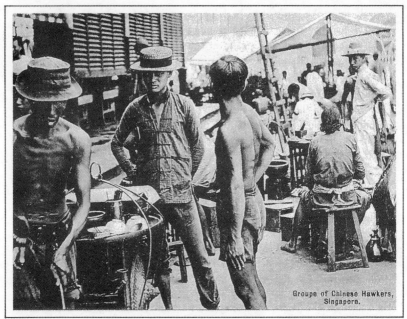

Groupe of Chinese Hawkers, Singapore.

GROUPS OF CHINESE HAWKERS

the bartering, the haggling, the odd burrowlike existence in narrow streets, the veiled existence of which we know, in any real sense, next to nothing. In the coolness of Singapore's short twilight you may recover again the charmed touch of the Orient.

"On the Empire Trail"
The Times, **August 9, 1921**

186

This Mystic Eastern City

"Travel has been my comrade; Adventure my inspiration; Accomplishment my recompense." With these words Charlotte Cameron summarised her approach to life. In 1921–22 she travelled 100,000 miles in the South Seas and almost immediately afterwards, embarked upon an exploration of Malaya, Borneo and Java, using Singapore as base.

A trip through the streets of China- and Malay-town . . . is intensely interesting. Rainbows of colour confront you on every side; you see how crowdedly they live – hundreds in a house; what feasts they are enjoying in their open-air restaurants on the pavement, obviously delighted with the – to us – most unappetising food. Their dried fish looks as if it must have been preserved since the days of the Ark. There are tentacles of octopus, bêche-de-mer, and little stuffed meat balls strung on sticks, which must form a happy hunting-ground for insects. Such messes! Such smells! And at some of the corners the pungent, nasty odour of the durian fruit, which they love, overwhelms all the other nauseous odours. Someone has graphically likened the taste of durians to that of an onion custard, poured through a gas-pipe, and seasoned with the hot, biting juice of garlic! Yet I heard an Englishman declare many times that he preferred durians to strawberries and cream! Surely there is no accounting for tastes. Durians are a large, green, rough-surfaced fruit with creamy-white contents. . . .

The Hotel Europe and Raffles Hotel are regarded as the best and the largest, while the Adelphi and Grosvenor are also first-class, but rather more of family hotels. Sea View Hotel is on the sea-front and is nice; there are many other smaller establishments.

The Europe Hotel faces the green lawns of the Singapore Cricket Club, and matches are in progress most afternoons, especially Saturdays. Here also are the football grounds, the natives taking a great interest in this essentially British game.

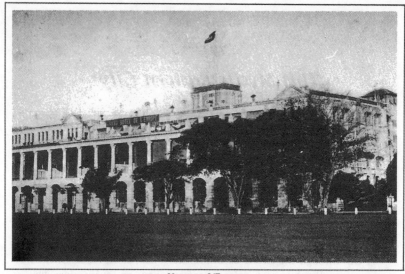

HOTEL DE L'EUROPE

A little farther on, facing the water-front, which is ever crowded with ships, is the large establishment known as Raffles Hotel. It has an open ballroom facing the sea, and is profusely decorated with gigantic palms. The entire hotel is surrounded by palms and trees, and here, twice a week, are held dinner-dances and dance-teas. The Europe Hotel has a large lounge with comfortable cane armchairs, always covered in white, and spotless, which creates an effect of coolness, ever welcome in the tropics. The ballroom is in the centre of the dining-room, the dance-dinner nights being Tuesdays and Saturdays. It is generally agreed that there is no choice between the Raffles and the Europe, both are good first-class, comfortable hotels, and the best you can find in the Orient. I stayed at the Hotel Europe. The tariff at either of these hotels cannot be regarded as moderate. For one room with bath, the price (food included) ranges from about $12 a day, or thirty shillings sterling. Inside rooms were $10, and suites naturally more expensive. Electric fans keep the place cool, and Chinese servants, always in white, are clean and attentive. The food is quite good enough. A curry, so beloved of the Easterner, is usually on the menu, and those who are partial to pineapples can surely feast, as this fruit is served at every meal, also bananas. . . .

Through influence I was enabled to see something of the night life of this mystic eastern city. Our party was first conducted to the opium-houses. In one large establishment with much gilding and marble on its front, there were four different floors, the higher being cheaper than the lower floors. Hundreds of Chinamen, well dressed in silks, were reclining on marble shelves and a hard wooden pillow on which their heads rested, and in their mouths a pipe. Holding a slender instrument resembling a knitting-needle, they would dip it into opium, make a small ball, twirl it over the flame of a spirit-lamp until the opium was sufficiently cooked, then put it in the pipe, and draw at it with blissful contentment. One wonders, yet dreads, what the after-effects must be. This was a smart "retreat" for the rich.

Afterwards we went into opium-dens for the poor – hideous, dirty, and smelly. Several Celestials were pointed out to us as being in about the last stages of opium poisoning. They become very yellow and emaciated, and will not eat; their one cry is for "dope" until the end.

As it grew late, one of our party suggested supper on the side-walk of a Chinese restaurant, daring us, in fact, to do it. We fell in with the suggestion, though our party included some officials and a lady of title. One of our friends, who was well known about Chinatown, selected a Chinaman whom he knew was dependable, and ordered some Chinese food for us. When we arrived, we had to sit on little low boxes close to the ground, whilst some shared a log between them. The light was very dim, but overhead a resplendent moon cast its radiant mystery around. In front of us were two braziers with red eyes, formed by holes punched in the iron to create a draught for the charcoal. Over these braziers some four or five Chinese were cooking *satis* for us. We opened our meal with bowls of rice, which we ate with chopsticks. The *sati* is composed thus: they take pieces, small strips, of raw chicken and twist them about a skewer, then twirl these skewers over the red-hot fire of the braziers until the chicken is grilled. They present you with a skewer of steaming chicken and two large bowls of sauce, one yellow and the other red. You are supposed to take the skewer from the Chinaman, dip it into the sauces, and then into your bowl of rice, eating it after the fashion of China. As soon as you had disposed of one skewerful of chicken, another was handed you. The red sauce was quite tasty, but the yellow pepper sauce made blisters on the tongue – it was absolutely painful. The chicken proved to be quite nice – dozens were served! Then came another problem: what should we wash the supper down with? The

189

only beverage obtainable was beer – and this without ice, eighty miles from the Equator. Well, I leave my readers to judge just how it tasted!

Never shall I forget Lady M ____ in evening gown, perched upon her overturned box-seat, eating *sati*, or the others all pretending they liked it, though really I don't believe they did. I have never cared for gastronomic mysteries, but it was a "lark," supping outside a Chinaman's shelter on the pavement, eating his food, the men of our party in evening clothes, and the glorious moon looking down upon a merry, irresponsible party.

CHARLOTTE CAMERON
Wanderings in South-Eastern Seas (1924)

1922

Strangers at Singapore

While travelling round the world, Charles Hendley, an American, wrote regularly to his son back in the U.S.A.

S.S. *"Melchior Treub"*
K. P. M. Line, Royal Dutch Packet Co.
Astride the Equator
SUNDAY, OCTOBER 22, 1922.

You may be interested in knowing what careful track the English keep of strangers landing at Singapore. Before we left the ship we had to have our passports examined by officers who came on board. As soon as we were registered at the hotel we were handed a circular to fill out, to be sent to some public official. We were required to tell on what date we arrived, from where we came, give our names in full, our nationality, tell what documents of identity we possessed, what was our profession, what would be the probable duration of our stay at Singapore, the probable date of our departure, and our destination. Then at the bottom of the circular in red ink was a notice that we should report within forty-eight hours to the Chief of Police, to whom we furnished about the same information we had given in the circular. I supposed I had done all that was necessary but on going to the office of the steamship company I found I could not go to Java until I secured permission from the Dutch Immigration Office, notwithstanding that my passport had been vised by a Dutch Consul. So I hied myself thither and after further questioning was given a white card permit and was able to buy my ticket and take passage for the "Gem of the East Indies.". . .

Singapore more than any other city is the clearing house for travelers. No matter from or to what ports the traveler comes or goes, from the Mediterranean to the Pacific, he must pass through the Straits upon which Singapore is situated.

There are some thirty languages spoken in Singapore, most of them dialects of the Malay and Indian races. These various tribes have imported not only their languages but their religions and their manner of dress and living. They all have dark skins of varying shades. What surprised me most was the extreme black skins of some of the East Indians. They are as black as any of our negroes and what startles one is to hear them (a few about the hotels) speak in clear excellent English. Many of them have fine clear cut features.

China has overflowed into all the countries about her. In Singapore, there are many Malays and Indians, but the majority of the population is Chinese. They make themselves at home in these neighboring countries and soon acquire a standing in business affairs. They are the real merchants of this part of the world. There are many rich Chinamen in Singapore and they live comfortably in expensive modern houses.

A story was told us by the American Bishop of the Methodist Church of these island possessions. One of the missions was planning to build, when they were offered such an unusual and excessive price for their ground that they accepted it. It developed afterwards that a rich Chinaman who had a home nearby discovered that at certain times of the moon the projected building would cast a shadow on his house and this would bring him bad luck; so he paid the price and kept away the evil spirits. The Chinese do not cater to the good spirits, saying that they will take care of themselves.

Of course the great mass of Chinese and Malays are very poor and live in squalid surroundings. In all these strange places that we visit I think I am more interested in the people and their customs than in anything else and the street life is always entertaining. In these hot countries the people live practically in the streets and all manner and grades of life are seen therein. All one had to do in Singapore to be thoroughly entertained was to watch the passing throng. . . .

The men as well as the women wear very bright colors, often vivid greens or reds or blues and there seem to be many different plaids especially in the *sarongs*. Some of the men wear long hair twisted in a knot on top of their heads or hanging down their backs unbraided. Most of them have smooth faces, but many of them are full bearded and some have rather fierce moustaches. It is startling to see a cart with two scared – excuse me, sacred oxen, and on top of the load a very swarthy man clothed only in a fierce moustache and a bright red *sarong*, his dark body glistening in the sun, whip in hand, urging on his patient slow steeds. The laboring classes do not wear shoes.

Of the more prosperous, nearly all dress in white, and to us it seems rather incongruous for a man to wear a well made and well fitting white duck coat, buttoned to his neck, and a plaid skirt and no shoes.

There are quite a number of Mohammedans among the inhabitants. Their religion governs many of their habits; among them the covering of their heads. They wear a turban or a cap like a fez.

We had a delightful drive through the Public Gardens and saw many tropical plants and trees. There were not so many flowers as the sun is too hot for them. It seems strange to find a golf course in a cocoanut grove and in fact there was a large hotel along the shore in the same grove. . . .

I had one unique experience. The Sultan of Johore was at the hotel, having dropped in on some business matter. I had the privilege of being presented and of having a private chat for a few minutes with him. He is a large, rather good looking man of about thirty-five, not very dark, and having been educated in England speaks English fluently. He said he had a number of American friends and was glad to see me. He remarked that Johore was worth seeing and suggested that May and I should go over and call on him which I promised to do.

CHARLES M. HENDLEY
Trifles of Travel (1924)

c. 1922

The Whitest Man in Singapore

Harry Foster, an American writer, was drifting through the East in search of material for a book. To support himself he took casual work; but Singapore and Malaya were then experiencing a trade depression and work was not easily available. Foster eventually found a job playing the piano in a waterfront bar.

Singapore at the moment was overflowing with human derelicts. Some were professional beachcombers. Some were well-meaning but weak-willed sailors who had missed their ships. Others were discharged employees from the rubber estates or the tin mines, for with the slump in rubber and tin – the principal industries of the Malay States – many better-class Europeans were finding themselves stranded. Nowhere in my travels had I ever found a city so full of the down-and-out as was Singapore at that particular moment . . .

. . . Chinamen filled the mechanical and clerical jobs, and the only employment for the average European was in some executive capacity, for which a drifting vagabond is not fitted. The whole scheme of the British was to maintain racial supremacy and prestige by employing white men only as managers. And these managers came out from home on contract. Even if there were a vacancy in some minor position, and a white man were willing to work for the same low wages as a Chinaman, the firm would not lower white prestige by employing him beside the Chinese.

Hence, in any British colony in the East, there were only two general classes of Europeans – those who were on top, and those who were on the bottom. There were many grades, of course, in the upper-class, and officials receiving three thousand a year would not associate with those receiving fifteen hundred, for a British colony is unsurpassed for snobbery. But there was no place for the tramp who would support himself by temporary employment during his wanderings, unless he happened upon a vacancy at the top and was capable of filling it, and such vacancies were scarce. If one did not come out on contract, to join those who were on top, there was only one place for him, and that was on the bottom. Just previous to my arrival, two stranded Englishmen had tried to earn a living by opening a bootblack stand; the Chinamen in Singapore were delighted at the opportunity to have their shoes polished by white men and began to flock to the establishment; the British officials promptly closed the place, informing the two English bootblacks that shoes were not being shined by white men in the Orient.

It is the only social scheme that would work in the East. No one values "face" or appearance more than the Asiatic. The Indians are accustomed to a caste system; the Chinese, when they become wealthy, love display; all Orientals are impressed by pomp and ceremony. The Englishmen aim to hold their respect by dressing like millionaires, riding about in automobiles or rikishas, stopping at palatial hotels, traveling first-class on steamship or railroad, and their system works, as I had early discovered when I tried to travel steerage back in Indo-China and was immediately ridiculed by all the Asiatic steerage passengers. The East is the land of "swank." Men and women who are nobodies at home will come out on some government position, and immediately begin to assume the airs of royalty. It is the only thing for the white man to do in the British colonies.

But if they can not do this, they must go to the other extreme, and beg for a living from their more fortunate fellows. Since beachcombers do not keep up prestige, the British government tries to send them home as quickly as possible, securing berths for them on British ships, and when this fails, even giving them a free passage on a passenger steamer. But at the moment of my visit to Singapore, the beachcombers were accumulating faster than they could be sent home.

Kwong, the proprietor, was a clever Chinaman. . . . he had gone to school, and spoke better English than nine-tenths of his patrons; although he was less than thirty years of age, he already owned an automobile and a handsome residence in another part of town; yet each morning at daybreak, he would be at the saloon, working in his shirt-sleeves or his undershirt, and would still be on the job at midnight when a Sikh or Malay policeman dropped in to suggest that the closing hour had arrived.

The Kid, as the nominal manager, strutted importantly about the establishment; Kwong, the real manager, stood meekly and quietly behind the bar, raking in the cash.

The Kid, although he made a valuable runner and publicity man in the morning, when he was quite likely to be sober, became more or less of a nuisance in the evening, when he was certain to be drunk. Then his old habits of bumming people would assert themselves, and even while he strutted from table to table, welcoming the guests, he could not check his impulse to borrow money from them, nor could he resist the temptation to sit down at any table where some one else was buying drinks for a group. The patrons began to resent his behavior, and not a night passed but some one threatened to "bash 'is bleedin' fyce in!". . .

Kwong had the Chinaman's aversion to physical violence, especially since such violence might result in the wholesale destruction of his furniture, and a possible loss of his license. He himself was constantly insulted by his patrons, who summoned him with, "Come 'ere, you bloody Chink!" but he concealed his resentment. Although in his intelligence and his manners he was infinitely superior to those who called him, he would come forward at a little trot and obey their commands with cringing humility. But after the last patron had been cajoled out into the street at closing hour, Kwong would send out for a large bowl of chicken, rice, and vegetables, and while the Kid and I sat with him and his bartenders over this midnight supper, he would sometimes express his real sentiments:

"Yes, Foster, I do not like to be called 'bloody Chink.' But that is the way of the White Man. If I were to resent it, I should lose his trade. And so I let him talk to me as Master to Servant. But all of his money, Foster, is coming into my cash-drawer."

Kwong's was the way of all the Chinamen in Singapore.

"Listen, Foster, according to statistics, less than five hundred Chinese paid an income tax this year, and yet I know for a fact that at least a thousand own automobiles. Believe me, Foster, these White Men whom you see at the Raffles or the Europe are not the wealthy men of Singapore; the millionaires here are Chinese, but they keep their wealth in the little Chinese banks almost hidden on side streets, and they do not make ostentatious display like the White Men. And many of these White Men here who live like millionaires, Foster, are posted at the clubs for not paying their dues or their gambling debts."

I read one day in a newspaper of a Chinaman who began life in the Straits Settlements as a rikisha coolie, and who, when he died in

Kuala Lumpur, left a fortune of nearly three million pounds. A Chinese sugar king in Java was reputed to be worth seven million pounds. There were many wealthy Chinese of lesser degree in Singapore, and some did live ostentatiously in magnificent homes, but most of them lived simply and obscurely, continuing to work meekly like Kwong, allowing the Europeans to strut about and put on the "swank," and profiting from the lordly, overbearing White Man.

Only once in twelve months did the Chinese observe a holiday, and that was on the Chinese New Year, which fell during my sojourn in Singapore on January 28th.

It was then that I realized how important were the Chinese in the industrial and commercial life of Singapore. The entire city ceased to move. Shops were closed. Ships could not be loaded or coaled for want of stevedores. In my Italian lodging house, which advertised a "French chef," my Italian landlady, like many another European housewife, was forced to cook her own meals, for even the so-called French chef, who looked suspiciously like a Chinaman anyhow, was celebrating the holiday. Only the very poorest coolies were at work – the rikisha coolies – and they were scarcely numerous enough to carry the wealthier Chinamen on their rounds of visits and calls upon relatives and friends. . . .

New Year is the great season for collecting or paying debts, and for giving presents; the Chinese, usually economical, are then in an extremely generous mood, and the Kid, who never missed an opportunity to approach any one in such a mood, came back to Kwong's upon the following day with fifty dollars in his pocket.

"S'easy if you know 'ow," he boasted. "A chink'll give you 'is socks if you know 'ow to talk to 'im."

All the other beachcombers crowded about him to demand the secret of such colossal success, and the Kid was not reticent about telling the story. He did not share the British national pride in keeping up white prestige, and he had gone begging to the palatial residence of the Honorable Eu Sing Tang, a wealthy Chinaman whose title came from an honorary position in the local government.

Hindu guards had stopped him at the gate, but the Kid had talked his way past them and into the private office of Eu. Inspired with unusual eloquence, he had pointed at the silken draperies of the apartment.

"Look at all them things!" he exclaimed.

Then he pointed at Eu himself.

"Look at your 'andsome, well-nourished body."

197

And finally he pointed to his own figure.

"And just look at me own skinny frame, and me unfed belly, and me ragged shirt. You're a Chinaman, Honorable, and you're a better man than I am, but you've mide your fortune from Europeans, and I'm a European. 'Ow about lending me a few dollars?"

The Honorable, like Kwong, spoke perfect English.

"Why don't you go to your own people?" he asked.

"Because, Honorable, I know that you Chinamen are the whitest men in Singapore."

That pleased the Honorable Eu Sing Tang. It flattered him, perhaps, to have a specimen of the lordly, overbearing race cringing before him. He called his servants, gave the Kid a bath in his own bath-tub, presented him with a new suit of white linen, fed him and gave him a glass of whiskey, and finally thrust fifty dollars into his hand, and bowed him from the house.

"S'easy," concluded the Kid. "Just tell 'im 'e's the whitest man in Singapore. 'E's a yellow devil, but 'e likes it."

There was an immediate exodus of beachcombers from Kwong's. They raced for the home of Eu Sing Tang. The Gorilla won the race, and when the Hindu guards sought to stop him, he floored one with a ponderous swing to the jaw, and rushed straight into Eu's private study. What transpired there I could deduce later from the Gorilla's story:

Eu looked up from his books and his ledgers with an expression of surprise and annoyance, but the Gorilla plunged into a repetition of the Kid's plea.

"Look at them heathen things!"

"Look at your fat belly!"

"Look at me, with a hole in me head and nothin' in me own belly."

Eu gave him the bath and the change of clothing, the food and the drink, but did not offer him the fifty dollars.

"Look 'ere," protested the Gorilla, "ain't you goin' to give me no money? They said you was the whitest man in Singapore, but you're the yellowest_____"

He could get no farther. Eu Sing Tang's servants seized him, removed the new clothes, threw him out into the street, and hurled his old breeches after him. He came raging back to Kwong's, accused the Kid of having deceived him, and gave the Kid a trouncing. The Kid, despite his many boasts, was no match for the little Gorilla, who dragged him out into the back yard where Kwong kept his empty bottles, and knocked him about the inclosure until it was a mess of broken glass.

Immediately three other bums, who had always wanted to lick the Kid, but had been overawed by the Kid's boasting, came rushing forward, demanding to be allowed a "go at the blighter." Kwong dissuaded them, and established peace by giving them all another drink, whereupon every one assured him that he, and not the Honorable Eu Sing Tang, was the whitest man in Singapore.

HARRY L. FOSTER
A Beachcomber in the Orient (1923)

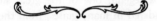

Then Entered Hamlet

"Native" theatre was one of the sights of Singapore, but seldom can these performances have received a notice in The Times *of London, as did this Malay version of Hamlet, enjoyed by a visiting* Times *correspondent and his friends.*

Shakespeare might seem somewhat remote from the cosmopolitan Asiatic community of Singapore, but, after a visit to the Star Opera House to see *Hamlet* performed by a Malay opera company to a mixed Malay and Chinese audience, one realizes that the poet is indeed not of an age but for all time, and one might add, for all countries. *Hamlet* has become a legend, one of the great stories of the world, appropriated and rendered in many guises, from the artificial simplicity of the new Reinhardt Theatre in Berlin to the cheerful pantomime of Malaya, where the actors' only link with the Western stage was the sight of an occasional Dutch rendering of Shakespeare in Java.

Notice having been given in advance that three white *Tuans* wished to attend a performance, *Hamlet* was chosen, after some discussion, as the most popular play in the repertory. The three arrived, to find a thoroughly Western and conventional theatre with elaborate drop scene, and seats as at home, except that the place of honour consisted of small boxes, like old-fashioned square family pews, immediately facing the stage. The curtain rose on a conventional room, from which a young lady in Western evening dress, attended by a small and solemn brown page, clad in becoming yellow cloak and cap like a Venetian picture, descended from the stage, with a tray of highly scented jasmine and tinsel garlands, which she hung round the necks of the embarrassed three amid the applause of the audience. There they had to hang till the performance ended, giving a finishing touch to the queer sensation of sight, sound, and atmosphere.

The players returned to the stage, and the first jolt was given to preconceived ideas by the discovery that the dark lady with inky hair was none other than the fair Ophelia, while the little page represented Horatio. The scenery and male costumes were interchangeable, it would seem, with those of *The Merchant of Venice* or *As You Like It*, giving a cheerful and sufficiently Shakespearian general effect of mixed colour. But the ladies had aimed higher, and the evening dresses and Western coiffures gave a curious air of a modern variety entertainment, while the Malay music and the curiously harsh voices (harsh at least to Western ears) suggested a pitch of up-to-dateness to which even our modern music has, happily, not yet attained.

The narrative of the past events leading up to the moment at which the play opens were performed in a sort of dumb-show, explained by chorus and recitative, and left no doubt in the minds of the audience as to exactly what had happened to the late King. Then entered Hamlet, unmistakable in his black suit, merely enlivened by some fantastic silver trimming which helped to harmonize him with his amazing surroundings. A fine actor, with the traditional conception of Hamlet's ironic humour, his contempt for his surroundings, and his bitter struggle with his own conscience, he dominated the stage whenever he was on it, and one felt, as one has so often felt when seeing other actors in the same great *rôle*, that the part of Hamlet is so created that it plays itself and the part creates the player, not the player the part. One felt the situation, the strife between the proud, sensitive nature and the cruel fate constraining it, through the grotesque surroundings and in spite of the almost unknown tongue, and, after a scene or two, the curious Eastern face, with reminiscences of Eastern sculpture and even a touch of the strange shadow faces of the shadow players of Java, seemed to be the Hamlet one has always known.

Hamlet himself connected this performance with the Shakespeare of all time, but the rest of the play was full of exciting surprises. The ghost turned out to be a comic character, introducing a scene of excellent burlesque in which the sleeping soldiers awake, and in the extremity of terror ring up the guardroom, and the corporal who answers the telephone, brave and truculent from afar, but the most abject of all at close quarters with the spectre, is an actor with a real comic gift, reminding one of certain French performers. There was all too little of this comedian, but at one moment, when the action flags slightly after Hamlet leaves the country, he reappeared in an admirable interlude of a white tuan (master) engaging a dhobie (washerman). His boy (servant) produces the dhobie and explains his qualifications, then the audience rocks with delight, as the master explains, in bad Malay, all that he expects in the way of service. At another moment, a small child entertains the house with a song and dance – very demure and very decorous, but making her exit with a wave of her hands and a look in her eye which bodes ill for her future career.

The scene changes to what seems to be the banks of the Seine, and, after a few more songs, the action of the piece is resumed, and the wicked uncle, more like the King of Hearts on a pack of cards than any real figure, is at last brought to his destined doom. Most of the great scenes of the play are given, but it is kept, in spite of the interludes, to a convenient length, and when one finally comes out into the crowded streets and the car makes its way slowly among the rickshaws and foot passengers, with the dim lights shining on the dark Malay faces and the shining smooth hair and bright ornaments of the Chinese women, it is with the feeling of a wonderful evening spent, which no one would have enjoyed more thoroughly than the divine William himself.

"Shakespeare in Malaya"
The Times, **May 1923**

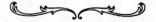

1923

The Shadow of a Woman

In August 1923 Mrs. E.F. Howell gave a talk to the Singapore Natural History Society on "Native Superstitions", based on her own experiences and observations.

At a meeting in the earlier part of this year, one of our members related a little incident which he had himself witnessed in front of the Victoria Memorial Hall; namely, the liberating from a cage, by a Chinese nonia, of a number of Java sparrows. As no one could explain the significance of this act, I made a few enquiries from a Chinese lady friend here, with the result that the following explanation was elucidated:-

"This custom is known as Fong Sang: a person having the idea that by releasing these living creatures, (birds, or fishes, that is), they will secure rewards in the world to come. It is a Buddhist belief, and is done in temples in Japan. The person was probably told at the temple that she might gain merit; or, the act was in mitigation for some sin; or, that she had promised if her prayer was answered, to let so many birds free."

Native superstitions and their significance surely form a most interesting subject, and as this Society includes ethnology in its branches, I am venturing to give a few experiences of superstitions, Chinese and Malayan, which I have come across personally in a residence of close on 20 years in Singapore, during which time I have found considerable pleasure, not to say instruction, in wandering about amongst the natives; trying, if I can, to glean even the tiniest insight on an outlook in life so different from my own.

The first superstition I came across was in connection with Kalangs, or fishing stakes. Over 18 years ago I was bathing with a party at Tanjong Katong. Being then as the Australians say, practically a "new chum," for I had had little time as yet to study the native, I begged to be taken out in an available koleh to see the fishing-stake nearby. My wish was granted, but as we were about to paddle alongside, the Chinese fisherman working on the stake, began to gesticulate and to shout out loudly in a very fierce tone. I was fortunate in my companion (a former Government servant, since, alas, killed in the Great War), in that he understood Chinese. But in reply to my query as to what all the fuss was about, he merely turned the koleh sharply about and paddled shorewards. When we were some distance away, he explained to me that the Chinaman had entreated him not to come near his fishing-ground so long as his boat contained a woman in it, seeing that even the shadow of a woman falling across his stake would bring him nothing but bad luck. . . .

The placing of a ring in the ear of a baby boy is a common practice among many natives, but especially, I have found, amongst the Chinese. Some time before I came to Singapore, a Eurasian mother whom I came to know later had had three daughters born, then two baby boys, both of whom died in quick succession. The sixth child being a boy, the anxious mother listened to the counsel of an old Amah, and a ring was placed in the infant's ear soon after birth. The boy survived, and holds a good position in Singapore today, whilst a fond mother and an aged Amah bless the little golden circle (still worn) which saved the child's life!

The obvious significance of this superstitious act is to "bluff" the evil spirits, who much prefer boys to girls. Great care must always be taken to lay the child down on the side which will expose the ear-ring, for the fateful moment is, usually, when the child is asleep. Then the evil spirits hover around, ready to seize their desire, but are baffled by the apparent symbol of girlhood. . . .

Almost every island in our harbour has its special kramat. There is one on little Pulo Hantu in Keppel Harbour, an island which bears the unpleasant reputation that any craft built under its shadow comes to an ill-fated end. On Pulo Kusut (the little peaked island opposite St. John's) there is a well-known kramat – the grave of a Malay – which is visited by streams of devotees on any free day, such as Sundays and holidays. This sacred spot is situated on the top of the peak, the way thereto being up some wooden stairs and the view over the harbour is well worth the climb. A Malay lives at the foot and ministers with rough courtesy to the pilgrims, who form a pretty sight, picnicking around in their gay garments.

It was therefore no surprise to me to hear that Pulo Ayer Mirbau possessed its own kramat. I had been over several times, however, before the Penghulu deemed me worthy of a visit to the holy ground. While treading the jungle path, the old rogue, garrulous as most Malays, told me that although he had been married to no less than 12 wives, (and divorced 11 of them), until eight years ago he had been childless. After marrying his twelfth wife, he adopted a small boy, seeing no hope of becoming a father. This, however, did not satisfy his wife (No: 12): so, like many a mother, from Hannah's day to our own, she determined to invoke the deity and plead "kurrat al 'ain" – "the joy of the eye" (as the phrase for a son runs in Arabic). Old Bakka pointed out to me the place of her pilgrimage, a small graveyard containing a few graves. Over one of these is placed a stone larger than the others, and over this stone he informed me his wife had placed a "white flag" tying it down with a piece of string to which an amulet was attached. (Such a sight is common any day in any Malay cemetery). The result was a happy one, for before the year was out a child was sent to gladden their lives, though the little one was the less-desired baby-girl. . . .

I have not yet discovered whether the Malay shares the Chinese dislike to a woman approaching a kalang, but one Malay superstition is not to throw the first fish caught into the bottom of the koleh. Wait until you have two, or you are liable to make a bad catch. Also to ensure success, spit on your bait before you cast it into the depths.

In February this year I came across a weird Malay superstition. I was about to step into my koleh at Pulo Ayer Mirbau prior to returning to Singapore one Sunday evening. The koleh was tied up near a Malay house, and as I placed my foot in the boat, a child in the house set up a plaintive wail. My boatman pricked up his ears, but his wife, a hardy old sea-dog who always took the helm, knit her brow and muttered something beneath her breath. The sea was calm, and the wind favourable for the return journey. However, soon after we had passed the tanjong everything changed: the wind suddenly altered its course and the sea uprose; from my wee koleh it looked mountains high, and for two hours we battled with the angry elements before we reached calm waters. And all the way, the old woman never ceased upbraiding the child whose untoward wail, just as we stepped into the boat, had wrought such dire effect on our home-ward trip.

Turning to building superstitions, these with the Malay are very elaborate, and much must be done to propitiate the gods of the soil before it is up-turned. That this had not been properly done when my small attap house was built was evident, for one Sunday when packing up to return to Singapore, I discovered a most unpleasant caller in the shape of a black snake. I immediately cried out for help, and the reptile – which measured about 4 ft. long – was quickly killed. I regret very much that my innate repulsion of the brute prevented my bringing over its corpse, or at least its head, as I should have done, to the Natural History Society.

When speaking to the Penghulu on the matter he took all the blame, inasmuch, he said, as he had set up the house in too great a hurry, and had failed to "propitiate the spirits of the up-turned soil.". . .

I think I shall be fairly in my province in referring to Love Charms as Superstitions. . . .

I had dropped in to see an Arab woman whom I have known almost since I arrived in Singapore. One evening when I entered her house, she was seated beside the bathing tank at the back of the common room, and standing beside her, each holding a tray containing culled flowers, were two younger women. The Arab woman breathed on the flowers, and made certain passes over them with her hands: the younger women then threw them into the tank. After waiting about a quarter of an hour, the Arab woman drew out two buckets of water therefrom and handed them to the girls, who turned and left the house, each bearing a bucket with her. It was explained to me that they were to bathe themselves with this water, and their heart's desire would come to pass. But the Arab woman added that if, when throwing the blossoms into the tank, any fell outside, the charm would be of no avail. . . .

Some years ago, a Malay jaga and his wife conceived a great affection for me, and on my return from New Zealand (in 1910), they were so overjoyed to see me again that they begged of me to accept a makanan besar from them and then to accompany them to a Mosque, where they intended to offer up a service of thanksgiving for my safe return. I accepted, and we sallied forth to the Mosque in Palmer Street, at about 11 a.m. one Sunday morning, the Malays bearing a dish of saffroned-rice and some ornamented hard-boiled eggs. I was not a little surprised that I, an infidel, should be allowed to enter in with these devout Muslims (I had, of course, to take off my shoes): I was still more surprised when the Imam beckoned me to him and, having said a prayer over me, proceeded to tie round my wrist a piece of yellow cloth. At that time cholera was rather prevalent in Singapore, and it was explained to me that while I continued to wear this band of cloth round my arm, I should be immune from it. Whether it was due to the charm or not, I cannot say, but I did not catch cholera either then or thereafter. . . .

This same jaga and his wife, not long after our visit to the Mosque, left Singapore for good, taking with them their three children. On bidding me farewell, the woman presented me with a small ring, containing five stones – so-called "diamonds" by the Malays – and explained to me that she gave it because neither she nor her husband could write to me of their welfare, or otherwise, in their own hand. But, she added, if any evil befalls us, look at this ring, for one or more of the stones will fall out – they represent my husband, myself and our three children. After about five months had elapsed, a strangely addressed envelope was brought to me by the postman. It came from an out of the way place in Java and, by the hand of a professional letter-writer, my friend Haji Abdul Karim enquired after my welfare, adding that he and his family were all well – only – the little baby had returned to the kramat of Allah.

On going home after work I examined the ring. The smallest stone had fallen out!

MRS. E.F. HOWELL
"Some Native Superstitions"
The Singapore Naturalist, 1925

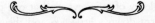

1926

Simply Wonderful

Edward Lane was travelling with some of his family on a world tour that was to last three-and-a-half years. He wrote regularly to his daughters back home in New Zealand, describing the journey in detail. These letters, including the following written at the Raffles Hotel, Singapore, were later published as a book.

Singapore is a most beautiful place, though I do not doubt that it has its drawbacks, if one lived here. It is hot, but not unpleasantly so, and the nights are perfect though one sleeps without bedclothes, except a sheet to lie on; and from what I can gather there is but little variation in the temperature the whole of the year. We have had a good look round, dodging about the island by car, and the roads are perfect – all bitumised wherever we have been. One day we went to Jahore and had a look at the Sultan's Palace and grounds – the latter very fine – also a large Mosque. We had lunch there and so back. The island is joined by a causeway, which is used by the railway as well as other traffic. Of course rubber plantations are everywhere – with cocoanut palms and pineapple plantations thrown in. Sunday morning we paid a visit to one of the rubber works where the crude rubber is fined for export. We also saw them collecting the milk from the trees, and it looks just like milk. We have also seen plenty of monkeys, and at one place where a temple had been; it was burnt down a little ago and they are getting ready to re-build. Monkeys are in a way connected with the temple, and we went provided with bananas; the old Priest, or whatever he was, called them and down they came, and Sharlee and Phyllis, as well as Mum, had great fun in feeding them. Some were quite tame. Of course there are all sorts of smells, and sights as well, and Chinese seem to predominate. The homes of private people are simply wonderful – and the gardens beyond description. You may imagine everything must look lovely, as Mum says she would like to live here. We have seen quite a number of

Chinese women with little feet, and it is wonderful how they get about. We saw an occasional one at Hong Kong, but here quite a number.

This is a very large hotel, and we have practically four rooms – a sitting room, bedroom, dressing room, and a bathroom. The lavatories are the funniest ever – no sewerage connection – but in the bathroom are two tripods with a seat, and of course, the necessary pan and a bottle of disinfecting fluid, and the man calls morning, noon and night. . . .

I think Mum and I are better off for clothes than ever we were in our lives. The white suits started with were about done, in fact I was reduced to one white jacket and two pairs of pants, so here I had some three suits made. I do not know what the stuff is called, but they are about the most comfortable suits of clothes I have ever had; and Mum had some frocks made. Hindoos are the makers, and it is wonderful how quickly they make them and how well. I am sure Mum has never had so little trouble with her frocks before. I also got a dinner jacket – had that thrown in as discount. So with the heavy clothes I brought from Australia I must have a suit for every day of the week. . . .

We have not seen a great deal of the city as one goes everywhere in rickshaws, so it is go where you want and return, though we have had a stroll round some of the streets close handy of an evening. It is funny to watch Phyllis Margaret – she does not like it a bit, and the way her nose turns up at the smells is funny. The pedlars are out of an evening selling all sorts of things, and the little push about cook shops, and the life that is on the streets is simply wonderful. Last evening we went for a stroll after dinner and stopped at a fruit vendor's to buy a pomella, and while trying to make the man understand, a tall native well dressed asked if he could assist, which he did, with the result that we got the pomella for 15 cents instead of 20. . . . There is only one drawback to this place, and that is the skeeters. We sleep in tents, and each evening before the boy closes them he has a hunt for the skeeter, but usually one or two hide, so there is another skeeter hunt when we get inside. . . .

Sharlee and Phyllis Margaret have gone with the man from Cook's to Sea View – a dinner dance there, also a swim. The bath is lit with electric light, and it will be ideal out there – a full moon also – so they should enjoy themselves. . . . While I think of it – while at the Club (Masonic) I met Captain D_____, who used to be in the U.S.S. Co., was on the Poherua and Pukaki about 15 or 16 years ago. It was quite a treat to have a chat with half a dozen Englishmen. I told a rickshaw man to take me to the Hall, and the man at the gate gave him instructions, but he got lost, so I asked an Englishman to direct him. He said if I had told

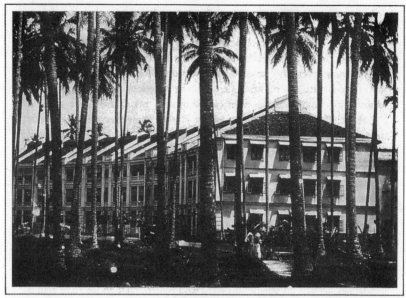

SEA VIEW HOTEL

him the devil house, he would have known where to take me, as that was what the natives call a Masonic Hall – rather a new name for it. Mum has shifted into the bedroom and is sitting underneath the fan writing away. . . .

Well, I will finish – we have had a happy time here, and it really is a most beautiful place.

EDWARD G. LANE
Letters written to my Children (1931)

c. 1926–27

A Sailors' Rendezvous

Alec Dixon came to Singapore as a police officer, and one of his duties was to examine the thousands of Chinese immigrants pouring into the Colony. Here he describes his work, his first impressions of the city, and his favourite restaurant, known affectionately to old-timers as the "Green Shutters".

To me, after seven years of close living in barrack-rooms, the police bungalow seemed luxurious. It was large enough to quarter a score of men, and my few belongings were lost in the wide rooms. The teak floors were dark with age and worn to a dull polish. White-washed walls and high ceilings preserved the illusion of cool spaciousness.

It stood on the threshold of Chinatown, backing on a busy main road which led to the docks. A front veranda overlooked the junction of five streets, four of which penetrated the heart of the Chinese city.

Except in rainy weather the house was shut up during the blazing mid-day hours; but after sundown doors and jalousies were thrown wide to catch the sea-breeze, and one could read or write in comfort. During my early weeks in Singapore I looked forward to the evening restfulness of those rooms, for there alone could I escape the urgent life and fierce colours of Asia.

I was puzzled by the strangeness of the city's skyline when first I saw it from the veranda of my bedroom; yet the explanation was simple: there were no chimney-pots.

Lines of tent-like roofs stretched from east to west. The corrugated tiles of the houses varied in colour from bright terra-cotta to greenish-purple, and faded, in the far distance, to a thin, metallic blue. An abrupt, palm-crowned hill dominated the roofs of the middle distance, its sheer slopes bloody in the evening sun. Scarlet and white banners flowered above the houses and marked that long, straight road which is the Oxford Street of Chinese Singapore.

211

Seeing that panorama for the first time, a stranger might well believe that he had arrived in China.

Travellers' palms stood like imperial fans in front of our bungalow, and their stems traced austere patterns against the yellow façade of a mission church. Although this building was dedicated to Methodism it was a splendid example of modern Chinese architecture. Its roof-points curved gracefully upward; and they were overshadowed by a square, pillared tower which recalled the serene beauty of the Forbidden City.

Through those green lattices I watched the unending pageant of the streets. Tamils, Javanese, Malays, Chinese, Siamese, and Sikhs – all Asia passed along that road. Their flesh-tints varied between old gold and sepia; and darkness turned them into predatory shadows. The constant mutter of their talk and the *clip-clop* of wooden sandals challenged the dull roar of the traffic. And on my first night in Singapore that tuneful clog-music lulled me to sleep.

Mohammed, our Malay gardener, spent most of his day in sleep, for he well knew that the garden would look after itself. Six healthy coconuts smothered one wall of the house and screened our southern veranda from the noontide sun. Ragged shrubs, flushed with hibiscus-bloom, fenced the compound on three sides.

The air of that garden pulsed with the stir of hurried propagation, for Nature was drunk with sunlight, and her bounty everywhere was lavish. The green of trees and shrubs never changed to bronze or gold with a dying year, for in that land was no winter rest, no springtime awakening.

After sundown the lighted rooms of the bungalow were open to the night, and privacy vanished. The shouting of bullock-drivers echoed in the bathroom. I shaved to the agony of a Chinese lament which drifted in from a neighbouring coffee-shop.

When the lights were doused insects appeared. First came the mosquitoes in wheeling flights to gorge on my fresh Northern blood. I heard their thin, angry humming as they side-slipped and dived hungrily at the hanging curtain. Then I turned my head to watch three inquisitive cockroaches explore the folds of a shirt. On the dressing-table a green mantis knelt like a huge grasshopper at prayer.

Only the lizards, ranging the walls and ceiling in search of insects, met with my approval, for they are welcome guests in a Malayan house. They are keen hunters, incredibly swift and silent in their killing. The Malays call them *chechak* – a word which sounds very like the noise they make in moments of exultation. They are translucent creatures about four inches in length, with eyes like tiny opals set in alabaster.

Bats of horrible size fluttered in like evil spirits, and outstayed their welcome. As I lay in bed I could see them hanging head downward from the ceiling fan – stealthy, loathsome creatures.

This menagerie dwindled before dawn, when the boy appeared, bearing tea and fruit. His coming heralded the most splendid hour of tropical day. Lying abed, with the mosquito-net raised, I watched the dawn blushing beyond a solitary palm which fretted the square of my window. Presently the black fronds turned olive, and then shone like silver spears against the clean sky of morning.

Once again the discord of a Chinese anthem reminded me that Asia waited on my doorstep. So, with the twittering of sparrows and rice-birds, the day began. Moments later I jumped out of bed and hurried to the bathroom. Already Fong had turned out the wardrobe, and was deciding what clothes I should wear that day. Never once while he was in my service was I permitted to choose the morning's tie.

In my bungalow was a bathroom which, had it contained a bath, would not have disgraced a Roman villa. The tiled floor sloped gently towards a grating which covered a small, dark hole. Near this hole stood a brown earthen-ware jar of remarkable design, large enough to accommodate the burliest member of the Forty Thieves. This had been filled to the brim overnight. A brass dipper, not unlike a lidless coffee-pot, dangled from a peg on the wall and completed the room's furniture.

After some deliberation I soaped my body from head to foot, and then, using the dipper, began a cautious baptism. The result was surprising: the water, which I feared would be cold and harsh, was as soft and pleasant as that sea-breeze which made the tropical night bearable. . . .

I did not immediately join the Mess at the bungalow for its members were all detective officers. As a new-comer in training at the Depot it was better that I should fend for myself. But the recurring menus, regular hours, and excessive charges of Singapore hotels put them out of a police officer's reckoning. My search was for some modest place near by; I had no car, and the constant use of rickshaws was expensive.

One day, by happy chance, a seafaring friend took me to a Japanese eating-house at Tanjong Pagar, which was scarcely half a mile distant from my quarters. This place was a surviving landmark of the last days of sail, and stood just outside the dock gates, where the road turned off to East Wharf. It was an old shop-house, solid but weather-stained with a signboard bearing Chinese characters and the name "TOKIO RES-

TAURANT" painted in shaky white letters on a green ground. The shutters of its barred windows, and a swinging half-door, gave it the appearance of a native liquor-shop.

Chinese beggars, emaciated and rheumy, cumbered the pathway. Dock coolies gambled and quarrelled in tight groups under the indulgent eye of a Sikh constable. Others stood, sat, or sprawled full-length before the door. The shafts of two rickshaws rested on the steps of the entrance while their pullers slept, open-mouthed, in the blinding sunlight. Flies settled on their lounging bodies, and, if stirred, spread in dark buzzing clouds to the offal of the gutter.

Tamil, Malay, and Chinese children played in the dusty road, careless of the heavy lorries which passed on their way to the docks. A light railway ran within ten feet of the pathway, and its Indian drivers made constant use of their heavy brass engine-bells. At the street-corner hawkers lowered their carrying-poles and stopped to chant the virtue of their wares.

Next door to the eating-house the forty-odd pupils of a Chinese school recited in a shrill sing-song for hours at a time. Yet despite its surroundings, the Tokio flourished, and in those days was known far and wide as a sailors' rendezvous.

The proprietress was a fat, middle-aged widow, built, as my seafaring friend remarked, on the lines of a Dutch brig. She was known to us as "Japanese Mary," and those who wished to air a smattering of her native tongue called her "Mamma San." She was no beauty, and the quality of her cooking rather than feminine wiles drew men to that house of the green shutters. Handsome or no, she was scrupulously honest and of even temper – a kindly, cheerful soul whose evening smile was as the morning.

Mary worked fourteen hours a day over her charcoal fire, while an ill-nourished Chinese boy trotted to and fro with dishes piled high for waiting customers. The Tokio's salads were the finest I have tasted east of Marseilles, and Mary's fish was the pick of the morning catch.

Sailors ashore demanded steak and onions garnished with crisp, brown potatoes – "Inglis staile," as Mary called it. With the smell of grilled steak in their nostrils, those sailors paid no heed to the story which the thermometer was telling.

Every day Mary set aside tit-bits for her regular customers. It might be lobster or salmon from cold storage, a tasty salad, or on special occasions a dish of her native *sukiyaki*.

Her few spare moments were spent at the back of the shop with her poodles, a bowl of goldfish, and a pile of needlework. Sometimes she would put in half an hour's work on the miniature garden which stood on the brick floor of the air-well. It was little more than four feet square, and she had collected its tiny trees and temples, one by one, during the thirty-odd years of her residence in Singapore.

In a moment of confidence she told me something of her history. As a girl of seventeen she married ("Inglis staile") the Scots master of a coaster running between Singapore and Banjermassin. Their married life was happy but brief, for he was killed on the bridge of his ship by a Malay who ran amok with a butcher's knife.

Long after his death, she said, the Tokio remained a kind of club for her husband's friends, for he had been a popular master in his day. Some of his contemporaries yet survived, and came with their friends to sup there on Saturday nights. Whatever the hour of their coming Mary never refused them. I have seen her turn to at midnight, without complaint, and cook a meal for six or seven lusty sailors.

Chinese labour was among the most vital of the Colony's imports, and Government steadily refused to check the steady flow of immigrants from China. Singapore was a free port in more ways than one. Any coolie who was able to crawl down a ship's gangway was allowed to land in the Colony on showing proof of vaccination. To pursue this century-old policy when China was in a state of chaos was neither wise nor practicable.

The only immigration law in existence was an ordinance which empowered the police to detain undesirable aliens within forty-eight hours of their arrival in the Colony, and if necessary to repatriate them. Such a law could be strictly enforced only by providing the port with a large immigration staff and a concentration camp on the Ellis Island model.

Concentration camps were regarded as un-British; also, they were expensive to maintain. The alternative suggested was that a police officer should board every coolie ship as soon as it anchored in the Roads. With the help of his Chinese detectives, he would weed out undesirable immigrants for further examination ashore. If after examination these appeared to be honest workmen they were to be released. If not they would be repatriated at the expense of the shipping company which brought them to the Colony.

Obviously the police officer chosen for this work had to be a detective of sorts. So it was that, since no other officer of the Bureau could be

215

spared, I was appointed Immigration Officer – temporary, acting, and all but unofficial – with a staff of two Cantonese detectives. My floating office was a twenty-foot motor-launch manned by three Malay constables of the Marine Police. The coolie passengers were inspected on board ships at the quarantine anchorage, about three miles from the shore.

Since I was, as far as I knew, the first Immigration Officer the Colony had seen, I was not troubled with annoying precedents, and my unconventional methods were not questioned. The work kept me at sea from dawn until sunset, and was very much to my taste. For several months I lived the life of a sea-gipsy, taking my food either at shoreside stalls or with the masters of the ships in the anchorage. Thus, I would breakfast with a Swede, lunch with a Dane, and dine with a Frenchman. . . .

Although they were young recruits my two Cantonese detectives turned out to be intelligent and reliable men with a remarkable aptitude for immigration work. Both were keen to acquire merit as detectives, and never once during those weeks at sea did either of them give the slightest cause for complaint.

The work of inspecting coolies was monotonous and very trying. Neither was it particularly pleasant. We spent many hours of the day breathing a stench so powerful that it fouled the air for two or three hundred yards about the ship. . . .

A few busy days at sea taught me to recognize the various types of coolie and to distinguish between workers and drones. It was my habit to feel the palms of the men's hands as they filed past the doctor, a trick which never failed to provoke laughter among the passengers. Nine out of ten of the hands I touched were hard and calloused. The tenth – a coolie with the soft hands of a cook – was invariably detained for further examination. This method was open to criticism, but it could be applied quickly – an important consideration when one was obliged to examine over a thousand coolies in the short period of half an hour.

The Mongolian faces of the coolies betrayed little or nothing. Gait, breadth and slope of shoulders, and depth of chest were safer guides to their owner's character and mode of life. Coolies of true peasant stock were easily recognized by their placid eyes and deliberate movements, characteristics of men of the soil all the world over. Yet it was no easy matter to pick out bandits and professional gunmen by such rule-of-thumb methods, for most of them lived hard, outdoor lives and looked as fit as any coolie or farmer.

Political agents, agitators, and teachers were more easily detected, since very few of them were of the muscular coolie type. One or two of these wandering intellectuals were lean and earnest youths from Shanghai who wore horn-rimmed spectacles and bell-bottomed flannel trousers. Most of the political agents were flat-headed Hailams, with smooth, sallow faces and shifty eyes. One of them invited deportation by addressing me, in an eloquent moment, as his "English comrade." These Hailams were inclined to be foppish in their dress, and invariably carried with them a good deal of luggage, which we searched carefully for incriminating books and pamphlets.

During my few months in the harbour I detained about three hundred Hailams. All but two of them wore what an English outfitter describes as "gents' boaters." I am not sure whether this is a coincidence or a psychological discovery; I state it merely as a fact.

ALEC DIXON
Singapore Patrol (1935)

c. 1927

Prison and Pork

As the headmaster of an English school in Kuala Lumpur, Richard Sidney showed perhaps a natural professional interest in another corrective institution while on a visit to Singapore.

Blue serge on police duty! It makes one sweat even to write about it. Not the police only: postmen, Government *peons* (messengers), prisoners themselves, all wear materials either made or made-up in Singapore prison. . . . If you see a cricket match played on coconut matting you may be sure that the matting was made at Taiping gaol or in Singapore; perhaps you need an easy deck chair for your voyage home – visit the prison and select one, they make them famously, in fact "the long lounge cane chair which is to be found so much in use all over the Far East was invented and perfected in the Singapore convict gaol."

Before taking you inside let me relate an incident to show you how differently the Chinese and the European regards imprisonment (for the latter it is disgrace and degradation, is it not?). . . . The gates of the prison were shut and safely outside was a close-cropped Chinese who had recently been one of His Majesty's guests: it was war time. The man looked regretfully at the closed doors – he seemed anxious to re-enter. Thinking the matter over he decided to try, and banged at the small gate. It was opened, and the warder seeing a recently discharged prisoner thought that the man had perhaps left something behind. It was not so: the released man wanted to go back! The warder was sorry; there was no re-admittance! The Chinese raised his voice and a few loiterers gathered near; as the man was being forcibly removed from the precincts they heard him say:

"There are numerous others who came in before I did; why shouldn't *they* be let out?"

There happened to come up to the Prison at this moment one of the

visiting Justices, and hearing the noise and seeing the crowd he asked
what all the trouble was. The matter was explained to him. In spite of
the War, prison dietary regulations had to be observed, these prescribed
so many ounces of pork per head. It was known that outside there was a
scarcity of pork. The Chinese preferred prison and pork to freedom!

It was a brilliantly sunny day, the time 1 p.m. when my friend and I
knocked at the small gate of Singapore prison, and immediately upon
entering were taken to the Chief Warder. Somehow I didn't feel as if I
was in a prison though all round me were evidences of the fact. . . .

"Better begin at the beginning," said our guide. "Here is the Office."

It might have been an office in any business house save for the clothes
of the workers, though I received a shock when I saw one whom I had
previously met in very different surroundings. This brought home
to me where I was and made me sorrowful. Except that his hair merely
bristled through his scalp and that he looked sad he seemed very
little changed. . . . We learned that no man who once entered was
likely in future to be able to escape detection. In the large ledgers,
arranged in a manner reminiscent of the catalogue room of Cambridge
University Library, was a complete record of each prisoner. There
were two mysterious initials "O or H." What were they? . . . They
stood for "Ordinary" or "Habitual." Next the room where finger-
prints are taken. . . . The process adopted is as follows, and I have
beside me the actual printed form used in this prison. It is divided
up into columns for the right and left hand, and our guide kindly
demonstrated how each finger after being coated with a thick black
mixture must be rolled from side to side so that at least three-quarters
of the finger's impression is recorded on the paper.

"But we are not content with these impressions only," added the Chief
Warder, "we must have as well the dab impressions of the eight fingers
taken simultaneously. And the clue is a good one, for not one person in
two millions has exactly similar markings."

We may imagine some prisoner, then, coming here after a gang rob-
bery and being entered fully in the record books and fixing his identity
by means of his finger-prints. For the first night he does not enter the
prison proper: he is weighed; must bathe and give up his own clothes
and put on a prison suit marked with red or black letters which denote
his term. In addition he will be photographed (such an interesting room
the photography room – the older camera having a Ross lens, and the
newer a Taylor-Hobson-Cooke), with his hands spread out flat on his
chest and with a mirror on the flank revealing his side face. He will have

a poor chance of escaping detection if he commits more crimes after leaving prison. . . .

We have seen already the Chinese ex-prisoner clamouring for re-admittance because of the pork; a visit to the prison cook-house when meals were being prepared makes one understand still more fully why many vagrants prefer the certainty of prison life to the hazards outside it. Here we saw that each separate race (at the date of my visit the prison population was Chinese 718; Malays 134; Indians 64; and Europeans 9) had a distinct portion of the cook-house. Chinese cooks were cutting up meat; white bread was being prepared for the Europeans' tea; and it was quite obvious that the three meals a day provide amply sufficient for the prisoner's nourishment. Everywhere, however, what I noted particularly – except in the Hospital – was the demeanour of the prisoners, they looked so cheerful and they were voluntarily working so hard – the European warders standing about having little to do so far as the maintenance of discipline was concerned. In the photography room, for example, were two long service criminals; but the keen way in which they showed me their newer camera, the obvious pride they had in their work, seemed to show that prison life was far from degrading them. It was the same everywhere else, and as we moved to another part of the prison and noted the vividly green grass contrasting so pleasantly with the sombre grey walls while above us the sun blazed from a lightly tinted blue sky, we seemed to be walking through some specially well organised factory. The illusion was deepened when we entered a large shed.

"In here," said our guide, "you will see many sides of our prison activities. Men on light duty making envelopes, others printing, others binding books."

But this was by no means all. Here were the tailoring and boot-repairing departments whose results we have already seen. Though they had no experts when either department started, yet very soon a specially good man emerged and he taught the others.

"Men serving a term of less than two years," said the Chief Warder, "are not taught a trade. They do the more unpleasant work of beating out copra. You'll see them later."

"And for how many hours a day do they work?" I asked.

"At present the regulations prescribe nine hours, but they would willingly do as much again. They hate being shut up!"

In another place we saw carpenters at work, one man was cutting out some balustrades. Others were making chairs – those long chairs which are so familiar in every bungalow throughout the East – with rattan tight bound round the wood. One special type had been designed by the wife of a recent Chief Justice and were known as "Lady Shaw" chairs. Herein, too, we saw stout wooden boxes being made – reminiscent of the play-box of schooldays. . . .

In the tinning department, no kerosene tins are wasted here, were being manufactured all the pots and pans for prison use. . . . Thence we walked to the looms – whereon towels, blankets, clothes and coir matting were being woven: to one who weaves a fascinating part of the prison factory. All the smaller looms had an automatic shuttle, so that the wefter could use both hands for beating up and his feet for pedalling. The Chief Warder was an expert in this department and told me that they produced more durable materials in the prison than they could buy outside. It was, however, the big loom weaving the material later on to become a cricket pitch that fascinated me. There were no fewer than eight men serving the monster. One stood behind the actual wefter and pulled the reed home after the gigantic shuttle, nearly two feet long, had carried the weft across the warp. Meanwhile others held the loom.

If the long-sentence prisoners are to be pitied we may at any rate feel that they are happily learning a trade, or practising one they know, and thus fitting themselves to hold their own in the world when they resume their place in it. But the short-term prisoners, serving less than 2 years, unless already qualified, are made to do hard labour – and as we moved to their open-air cells we could hear the rhythmical hammering note which indicated that they were beating out copra. The hammer on the husk of the coconut shell sounded quite pleasantly musical. Before these husks become the coir rope which we saw being woven they need to be soaked for many days; the water in the tank is never emptied but merely added to from time to time – at one end its colour was a deep red showing how the coconut husks had absorbed all they could, at the other end it was nearly clear. The water has the effect of strengthening the coir. Lying about were broken coconut husks from which after much beating was extracted the stringy substance which after separation into strands is wound together and made into rope. The men were working each in a separate cell and had to beat out a specified number of pounds per day. Most of the cells were open, a few were closed, barred and padlocked. Inside were prisoners who had been detectives and whose presence was resented by the others: they were locked up for safety.

Besides these places we also visited the segregation cells where men awaiting deportation – banishees – and lunatics were housed temporarily. One poor fellow, quite naked, convinced that he was a famous dancer, performed as soon as his cell door was opened. Every now and then he banged himself against the smooth wall of his cell – but otherwise his exhibition was graceful and his movements skilful.

The condemned cells were, to me, the most dreadful part of the whole prison. Luckily they were empty. . . . The Governor of the Prison, although he kindly allowed me to hear full details of all the grim details of the condemned man's last moments, asked me specially not to publish these. I can say, however, that the process is as humane and as skilfully performed as anywhere in the world. . . .

But away from gloom. . . . Come with me to the quarter wherein live the criminal ladies – not very many; and it is astonishing how few are the women prisoners throughout Malaya. Of course the women, too, misbehave. Only recently a well-dressed Chinese lady, carrying an attaché case, asked to see the Protector of Chinese (or as it was called in that town – the Secretary for Chinese Affairs) and was shown into the Office where the European Officer was sitting at his desk. She began to speak and as she did so fumbled with the lock of her case. . . . Outsiders heard a loud explosion, and when a clerk came rushing in he found both European and Chinese badly wounded by an infernal machine which the "lady" was carrying in her bag. Both, I believe, recovered. So you see prisons have to reserve some space for women offenders. One lady we met was serving her second "life" sentence the Chief informed us.

"Yes," said he, "she looks quite pleasant and harmless, doesn't she? and she behaves admirably I am told." Here the matron nodded. "And yet," continued the Chief, "that woman did 15 years for one murder, and after being let out promptly killed somebody else. We shall have to keep her here now."

RICHARD J.H. SIDNEY
In British Malaya Today (1927)

1931

An Eastern Petticoat Lane

R.N. Walling, who worked for the Singapore Free Press, *had the idea of turning what he called "the provocative light of modern journalism" on to areas of Singapore life. Here he turns his spotlight on a colourful corner of the business district – Change Alley.*

It is easy to pass by without noticing Change Alley, at either end. The unprepossessing wooden archway opposite Collyer Quay effectively conceals the glamour that lies beyond and acts as a barricade against the confused babble that rises like a lot of hot air inside.

It cannot be much more than a hundred yards long and, as if guarding jealously its business secrets, both ends are quiet and sleepy.

I "dived" into Change Alley – as delighted American tourists would no doubt like to describe their entrance into this shrouded thoroughfare to those "way back" – somewhere about noon, at the height of the day's business. In a city the cosmopolitan inhabitants of which reveal little of their true environment, the dense crowd of Jews, Arabs, Chinese, Japanese, and Indians, bartering and selling in an atmosphere cool in comparison to the tar-macadam roads outside but delightfully stuffy, smelly, and dirty, really, was invigorating and faintly exciting.

. . . the noise of the hawkers of fountain pens from Germany, socks and silks from Japan, ice-water, toffee sticks, fruits, shirts, pants, scissors, pencils, nails, curios, and the thousand and one necessities of Asiatic life and existence; the shuffling of many feet, the panting, the breathing, the spitting: the "shop" of Chinese produce dealers, commission agents, unguaranteed brokers, and compradors to European firms – kept up the incessant glamourous din of an Eastern Petticoat Lane.

On each side of the alley, retailers by the dozen had set up in business; dark, dingy stairways leading to Asiatic lawyers' offices, barbers' shops, and eating places besides – it is amazing how much activity is packed

223

into this confined space. There must surely be more business per square foot in this alley than anywhere else in Singapore.

About the only place in Change Alley that carries with it the more or less dignified Mincing Lane atmosphere of yesterday is the exchange market frequented by Chinese produce dealers; dealers in Gambia (Java, Hamburg and Press cubes), Singapore and Muntok white pepper, mixed black pepper, sundried and mixed copra, tin, small flake tapioca, and medium and small pearl, No. 1 sago flour, and "Borneo" "Palembang Jelotang" "Banta" and "Sarawak" (whatever they mean!).

Here everybody sits and reads Chinese papers at a long deal table, in an atmosphere of pepper, sundried and mixed copra, small flake tapioca – but mostly smoke! People are always strolling in and out, and every now and again someone gets up from the table, nods, and goes into one of the rooms at the back to sign a contract. He has probably been arguing with someone for half an hour or so at that long deal table – reading papers!

It's like an auction room without an auctioneer.

While all the time an anxious secretary stands by a blackboard, with an imploring look in his eyes, waiting to mark up a buyer and a seller. It is hard in these days to fill in all the spaces. I half expected someone to give a cheer when he started putting figures by the side of Muntok white pepper and copra, but apparently they've been doing quite well lately.

Ten years ago Change Alley had a name which was well-known in business circles in London and New York.

Millers met the commission agents dealing in raw rubber from the outstations; bought, and sold again through the European agents to the European consumers. In those days there was only one guaranteed broker. Now that there are three, not to speak of a whole host of unguaranteed men, business is mostly transacted over the telephone – and Change Alley has changed from Mincing Lane to Petticoat Lane.

Once it was of first rate importance in the business life of Singapore – now it is only second rate.

It is a sign of the times. Ten years hence, or less, Change Alley may no longer bare this Municipal notice at the diminutive entrance from Raffles Place:– "No Hawkers are Allowed to Ply in This Street." Or, no doubt, it will, and it will no longer strike me as funny!

R.N. WALLING
Singapura Sorrows (1931)

1934
Monsoons and Sumatras

Singapore's weather is an ever-interesting topic but one not well understood by passing travellers. This extract, therefore, is from a third-generation resident and member of a distinguished legal family whose Singapore origins go back to 1862. Roland Braddell introduces two "very welcome visitors", the monsoons.

In Singapore the weather is like that of every other place – most unusual for the time of the year; and we generally blame it on the monsoons. "It's between monsoons" or "The monsoon hasn't broken yet" or "The monsoon is very late this year"; you'll hear plenty about it in these parts. It is important for you to know about these winds, for they affect one's comfort very materially.

The word is derived from the Arabic *mausim*, meaning season, and a monsoon is a seasonal wind caused by the summer heating of the land masses of Asia and then by their winter cooling. There are accordingly two monsoons: the south-west or summer one, blowing from May to October and the north-east or winter one, blowing from November to April. At the end of each there is a very wet period of about one month when the winds are light and variable. Singapore is so near the Equator that the monsoons have quite a different effect from what they have in India. The south-west is hardly felt at all; the north-east, though much stronger, in nothing like the ferocity which it displays in the Gulf of Siam or the South China Sea; but both are very welcome visitors. The north-east is the cooler one, bringing plenty of rain and lots of cold nights; it is then that the big round-the-world tourist ships come, and the ordinary liners give forth their full quotas of visitors. Singapore always wakes up in the north-east monsoon, and the hotel people and the shopkeepers grin round the town like the dogs of the Psalmist. . . .

In Singapore we get no typhoons or cyclones and no earthquakes; our only abnormal unpleasantnesses are violent squalls of wind and rain.

These come only during the south-west monsoon, and we call them "Sumatras," because they are caused by the monsoon being obstructed in its course by the mountains of Sumatra. The wind during these squalls, which frequently cover a front of as much as three hundred miles, usually comes from a south-west or westerly direction and is invariably accompanied by blinding rain, making navigation in the Straits of Malacca extremely hazardous. Ashore the wind and rain blow with fury against the houses, so that, if one's windows and doors are not shut tight, Aunt Mary's photograph is blown from one room to another, the curtains stand out at right angles, and falling objects beat a tattoo everywhere. The whole thing, however, passes as quickly as it comes, and the "Sumatras" are well understood, giving plenty of warning to the wise that they are on their way.

Our "terrible climate" is in reality quite a reasonable one, though enervating. May and June are the most disagreeable months, owing to the prevalence of the southerly winds which we call "Java winds." It is remarkable that the stronger these winds blow the more enervating they are, and this is particularly noticeable at Katong on the seacoast. They also generally bring colds and minor fevers, particularly influenza and dengue, so that the Malays call them expressively *angin jehat*, or evil winds.

It is seldom, at any time of the year, that the mornings and nights are not cool, since diurnal breezes from land or sea blow over the island. The afternoons between half-past two and four o'clock are usually very hot. Mean temperature in the shade through the year is about 81°.5 F. The highest to which the shade thermometer is liable to go is 90° F. and the lowest 73°.5 F.

ROLAND BRADDELL
The Lights of Singapore (1934)

c. 1934

A Most Amazing Adventure

Robert Foran was a journalist-traveller, commissioned to spend six months in the East, motoring through British Malaya and neighbouring countries to record his impressions.

On my first day ashore in Singapore, I was under the impression that some great national or religious festival was being celebrated in the Chinese quarter of the city. From the upper windows of the houses in these streets densely populated by Chinese, I could see suspended long bamboo poles, each one being profusely decorated with a confusing array of multi-coloured cloths. The blue of China – everything seems blue in China! – largely predominated; but an age-grimed white ran it a fairly close second.

Inspection at near range, however, revealed that the articles fluttering in the breeze above my head were no more than wearing apparel. . . . Even if it did somewhat mar the fading beauty of these quaint Oriental streets, yet necessity is the mother of invention. The harassed mothers of large Chinese families, who lived in those crowded tenements, had no back gardens available for hanging out their washing to dry. As all Chinese garments are of the same square-cut shape, it is simple to pass a bamboo pole through the wide sleeves or trouser legs, thus exposing all of the article to sun and wind. This plan dispensed with lines or clothespegs. . . .

Singapore's streets are always seething with life. The noise is indescribable. London, New York, Paris and other great cities are bad enough; but they are a haven of peace in comparison with Singapore. The Malay drivers of motor-vehicles have a failing which is highly objectionable. The horns or buttons of the mechanical hooters on cars and lorries prove quite irresistible to their childish minds. Their itching fingers are never off them for more than a few seconds at a time. They behave exactly like infants provided with a drum or cornet to amuse themselves,

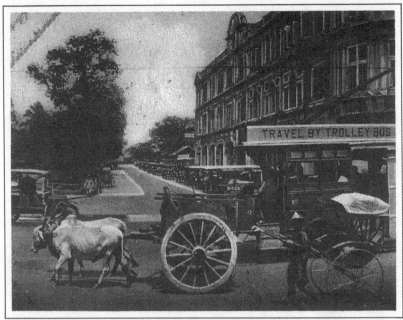

LOCAL TRAFFIC

and make full use of this golden opportunity to render life hideous for others. It does not matter in the least to these native drivers that there is no real occasion to give warning of their approach. They argue that the hooter was provided for use, and are not niggardly in sounding it. They are an infernal nuisance in the city's streets, for they create Bedlam by day and night.

Frequently I saw a long row of taxis on a stand, and each driver was entertaining the neighbourhood with his share in a motor-horn symphony. Some sat upright, putting heart and soul into their contribution to the cacophony of sound; others smoked cigarettes and lolled back in their seats, while keeping *their feet* pressed heavily on bulb or button. The noise produced by this amateur jazz-band can best be imagined than described. It must have been a nerve-racking experience for the occupants of adjacent offices, even as it was for those who passed through the street. The constant sounding of a dozen different varieties of motor-horns and buzzers cannot be recommended as a musical entertainment.

228

Sleep at night in the hotels, until you grow accustomed to this inflic-
tion (if you ever do), is practically an impossibility. Until two or three
o'clock in the morning this hellish nightmare never ceases. Two hours
later, the obliging church-bells of the city begin to toll forth their sum-
mons to prayer, while the impromptu symphony of the motor-driver's
orchestra is resumed with renewed vigour. Three to four hours of sleep
at night was about as much as I managed to get during the first few days
in Singapore. In such a climate, this can lead only to the grave, murder
or a lunatic asylum.

While I was in Singapore, a Dutch girl had a most amazing adventure,
and escaped death only by a miracle. She was a passenger on a Dutch
liner to Batavia, which left Singapore about ten o'clock at night. The
girl went down to her cabin soon after the steamer left the docks,
intending to go to bed at once. She had the cabin to herself. When
almost undressed, the beauty of the lights of Singapore attracted her
interest and she leaned out of the square port-hole to view them better.
At that moment the ship suddenly changed her course eastwards, and
gave a violent, heavy roll in doing so. It caught the girl unawares.
Before being able to save herself, she slipped out through the port-hole
into the sea head first and clothed only in silk underclothing. As soon as
she came to the surface, the girl started to shout shrilly for help. Her
cries were not heard on board. Soon the vessel had left her far behind
and was fading from sight. Terrified, she started to swim and float in
turns, hoping that some passing boat might see and rescue her. As it
happened, the girl had only learned to swim about four months earlier
in Holland.
Throughout the long hours of that dreadful night she managed to
keep afloat, heroically refusing to give in. Her terror was increased by
the knowledge that the waters were alive with sharks. Fortunately,
though strange fish occasionally bumped into or brushed past her, no
shark appeared or attacked.
Just as the dawn appeared, two Chinese fishermen saw her and rowed
over to where she was swimming spasmodically. They hauled her on
board, giving her water to drink and some boiled rice to eat. The girl
could not talk any language they knew, or even understand what they
said. By signs, she tried to persuade them to row back to Singapore; but,
with callous indifference to her plight, they shook their heads and
resumed their fishing.
All through that terrible day, the wretched girl crouched down at the

bottom of the boat, subjected to the full rays of an Equatorial sun and with no covering to protect her save the filmy silk underclothes. The terrible sun burned, scorched and blistered her whole body, the effect being infinitely worse owing to the salt soaked into her skin from the sea-water. She suffered unspeakable torments. At times, she told me afterwards, consciousness left her; at others, she shivered to think what the Chinese fishermen might do to her. Throughout that day the sun blazed down upon her, burning and blistering her semi-naked body from head to foot.

At long last, just before sunset, the fishermen started to row back to the harbour. By this time the girl was unconscious and in delirium. When they reached the harbour, the fishermen reported the circumstances to the nearest police-station, and prompt action was taken. It chanced that I was motoring past the police-station, and my car was impressed for duty as a temporary ambulance. Wrapping her carefully in a rug, we made her as comfortable as possible on the back seat and drove rapidly to the European hospital. Doctors and nurses instantly did everything possible for the patient.

It seems an incredible tale, yet it is perfectly true. I heard the full details of that ghastly night and day adventure from the girl's own lips in hospital, as soon as she had recovered sufficiently to receive visitors. There could be no doubt as to the truth of her statements, for most of her body was swathed in bandages as the result of the long exposure to salt-water and a tropical sun. How she managed, a weak and inexperienced swimmer, to keep afloat all through that dreadful night, she could not tell me. "I was not intended to drown," she smiled at me.

The age of miracles is not yet dead!

The road out to Sea View does much to spoil the delights of this popular resort. You must proceed via Beach Road, and through a barrage of smells of infinite variety and nauseating qualities. There is only one other route available – a drive by a circuitous road, which takes you half-way round the island. Notwithstanding, many Europeans and wealthy Chinese dwell at Tanjong Katong, and drive twice or more each day through a series of smells such as rival even the Singapore River at its worst. They are either long-suffering or foolish! If you could escape the pestiferous evil of that drive to and fro, then Tanjong Katong (or Sea View, call it what you like) might be written down as a delightful asset to Singapore. As it is, the approach entirely kills its many charms.

Starting from the centre of the city by way of Beach Road, it is well to adjust your gas-mask or handkerchief to the nose. The first odour to overpower you is the strong fishy smell from the Clyde Terrace Market. This, however, is *Eau de Cologne* compared to what will follow in rapid succession. Take heart, if you can, for it is only a five miles drive to Sea View.

Comes then a most objectionable aroma from the drains in the native quarters, which are used for all kinds of insanitary and wholly unauthorized purposes in addition to draining the livestock shops in Rochore Road. Next the powerful stench from a number of rubber and pineapple factories assails you forcibly; and follows a strong gas attack from the Municipal gasworks. The latter are situated in Lavender Street. Was this unconscious or deliberate witticism, or merely a touch of subtle irony? Whoever was responsible for the naming of this street had his little joke!

Then envelop you the smells emanating from still more rubber and pineapple factories, quickly rendered ineffective by the powerful and sickly effluvia from the fever-laden mangrove swamps close to Sea View. That drive offers no pleasing prospects either going or returning – nasally speaking.

Once you are through this dreadful barrage of smells, Sea View has much to offer in compensation for all endured in getting there. The sea-bathing is really first-class, the air refreshingly cool from ocean breezes, and you can lunch, tea or dine on green lawns while listening to the rhythmical boom of the breakers. The star-decked canopy of the night is your roof for dinner, and the nodding plumes of palm-trees your background. Sea View always struck me as an ideal place – once there; but, at the back of my mind, always lurked the terror of that drive back to Singapore.

W. ROBERT FORAN
Malayan Symphony (1935)

1934

The Daily Double

Douglas Graham and his wife had become friendly with the Cowlings – who were Singapore residents – on the boat out, so they were well entertained during their stay in town. Graham afterwards published his diary of the trip "so that our children and grandchildren may be inspired at some convenient time to go and do likewise".

March 1st. Quiet day. Played Bridge against our last night's opponents and repeated our victory, but this time winning nearly three guilders each. Arrived 10 p.m. in the harbour of Singapore. Very hot in cabin – 84°.

March 2nd. Left boat at 8.30 a.m. for Raffles Hotel, which is a big place but not particularly luxurious. Nice big bedroom and bathroom. After a drive round, lunched at the Hotel with the Cowlings and their sister and their recently married niece. Also Mr. Cowling's father, a very entertaining old man, who was once a Director of Education in the Malay Peninsula. Speaks 15 languages.

At night dined with the Cowlings at a Chinese restaurant. This was a very big place. We were shown into a private room by two Chinese well known to the Cowlings, and who dined with us. Were waited on by three Chinese girls. After drinks – whiskey and beer – dinner was served. It was the weirdest I had ever had. There was bird's nest soup, sharks' fins, the skins of pig and duck, the latter two served with various sauces. At intervals one of the girls discoursed music, singing to a zither played with a bamboo hammer. All the songs were sung *piano*, and sounded very sweet only what the words indicated I haven't the slightest idea. I was informed they were love-songs.

Then went up a lift to the top floor, where we found ourselves in a Chinese theatre. A play was being performed. The audience was 100% Chinese until we appeared. They sat in no regular order on little stools round the stage, with a constant movement. It was a most

232

unusual and intriguing scene to me. Chinese men, naked to the waist, others in immaculate European clothes, mixed with their women kind, some carrying babies. This was the Cantonese theatre.

Later, after partaking of a cup of coffee we descended to the next floor where there was a similar crowd, only a different style of play, peculiar to Shanghai, was being performed. It was most fascinating. The stage is really a platform, and has no wings, only a back-cloth. The stage hands move about the stage altering the scenery while the actors are performing, and they are always visible. In the Cantonese theatre the costumes were hung up at the side of the stage and taken down as wanted.

Afterwards we adjourned to our private room on the second floor where we partook of more drinks and sweetmeats and fruit. The oranges were particularly sweet and luscious.

Smoked a pipe of opium but experienced no sensation.

March 3rd. In the morning drove to two golf courses, the Singapore and the Island. Both are most beautifully situated, so fresh and green, with a reservoir in the middle. The Singapore is entirely European, but the Island is mixed. I was told the Chinese were quite experts at the Royal and Ancient game. In the afternoon lunched with the Cowlings at their bungalow.

Afterwards they took us to a meeting at the Singapore Racecourse, which, it is claimed, is the finest in the world. This statement I took with a grain of salt, but after seeing it I felt sure the claim was justified. The grandstand is of noble proportions, three-tiered with lifts. All the seats are cane-bottomed and most comfortable. The course lies in front, oblong in shape, the far side is on the side of a hill, so one can view the races from start to finish with the greatest ease. The stand is double-sided. At the back are wide open verandahs on which are the totes both for paying in and out, the tea cafés and the bars. The view at the back overlooks the car park and main entrance, and, what is more important, you have an excellent view of the huge tote indicator. In fact, you see everything without leaving the stand.

There are several lawns of beautiful turf. The judges' box is opposite the centre of the grand stand and there is a huge clock with a hand at least six feet in length. At the moment of the race this hand revolves, and stops when the first horse passes the post. The exact time of the race is then exhibited clearly. On the right-hand side of the judges' box is the saddling enclosure, also plainly seen from any part of the stand. Alongside of this enclosure but on a level with the stand is the weighing-in room.

All the betting is done on the tote on a 4 dollar unit basis. There are 24,000 members and no one is allowed to bet unless he or she is a member. We were made members for the day. There were nine races on the card. Horses, as far as I could judge, were really first-class. Everything was convenient and really luxurious.

The crowd were practically all in the grand stand, and what a pretty picture they made – so cosmopolitan – the well turned out European lady contrasting with the Asiatic Chinese lady with her slashed skirts, showing one leg at times quite freely, and the dainty Japanese in her best kimono.

Our host, Mr. Cowling, had a horse in the last race. It was second favourite, but, alas for our pockets, did not catch the judge's eye at the winning post. The race card was the most complete one I have ever seen. Besides the usual card for the meeting, it also contains a guide to the form of the horses running and other information. It is issued in a very handy form. Finally the car park arrangements are perfect, like everything else connected with this ideal course. The whole course and buildings cost over a million pounds to build.

I noticed as I went out, exhibited on a large board, the amount of the Daily Double. The first prize was over 53,000 dollars, and there were other prizes in addition, and this on the third day of the meeting, which gives one an idea of the magnitude of the betting.

In the evening the Cowlings took us to a Japanese restaurant. This was some miles out of Singapore and was pitched by the side of the sea, the wooden building being on piles in the water, so one had to cross a bridge to enter. The first thing on entering we removed our shoes and stood in our stockinged feet. We were met by four Japanese girls who conducted us to a room overlooking the sea. The room was practically bare of furniture except for a low seat round it. After drinks were served – again beer and whiskey, the latter being unusual and for our special benefit – a low table was brought in with a square hole in the centre. In this was placed a charcoal brazier. A large plate of piled-up uncooked fish, meat, etc., was then produced. This was cooked on the brazier while we all squatted around. Chopsticks were handed round. Our soup basins were piled with rice and on another plate we helped ourselves from the concoction in the centre when it was cooked. This was eaten by the aid of chopsticks – at least by the other guests. I was so inexpert at the game of picking up minute grains of rice with most inadequate instruments that the Japanese girls took pity on me by giving me a spoon and fork. I got on well with these modern feeding implements. I also was allowed to recline instead of squatting, the correct mode, and in addition was favoured with several soft cushions to protect my bones from the hardness of the floor. Saki was served warm in tiny saucers and I found it quite pleasant to taste.

After dinner we sat on the settee round the room, with a full moon shining in from over the sea making an unusually pretty picture. The girls, four of them, gave us a dance, accompanied by music played on a zither. The dance depicted by action and song the sowing and reaping of rice. Mother enjoyed this show much better than the Chinese one the previous night. She was quite handy with her chop sticks and ate her food and drank her Saki with gusto and satisfaction.

Returned to the hotel, and after liquid refreshment bade goodbye to our charming and generous hosts.

J. DOUGLAS GRAHAM
My Wanderings in the Far East (c. 1935)

1936
Secret Shame

As a young man, Bruce Lockhart had been a rubber planter in Malaya. Now after an absence of twenty-five years – during which he worked as diplomat, writer and journalist in Moscow and London – he returns to find Singapore much changed.

Thirty years ago ... legalised or semi-legalised prostitution flourished throughout Malaya. Indeed, eighty years ago vice was so rampant that, rather than allow ship's crews on shore, foreign Consuls in Singapore and in other East Indian ports used to arrange for boatloads of inspected prostitutes to be sent on board for the duration of the sailors' stay in port. Even in my time Singapore deserved a certain reputation for vice. The vice itself was never at any time so lurid or so glamorous as it is still painted by certain travellers and by the scenario writers of Hollywood. The reputation may die slowly, but now it is certainly not deserved. Here, too, change has worked a minor miracle.

Singapore was the first city in which I had ever seen at first-hand the sale and purchase of vice, and the temptation to revisit what had then seemed the street of adventure was irresistible. Accordingly, just after sunset on the evening of my third day I ordered my chauffeur to drive me to Malay Street and Malabar Street, where formerly the white wrecks of European womanhood and young Japanese girls, silent, immobile and passionless, traded their bodies for the silver dollars of Malaya. As I drove down the beach front, the lights began to appear on the ships in the harbour like so many little lives which would vanish in the morning, for Death is still an early caller in these tropical parts. There was the faintest of cooling airs from the sea. By the time I reached Malay Street it was already dark.

I had chosen this hour intentionally for my attempted recapture of the spirit of a past which had eluded me ever since my arrival. Recognition returned with a momentary thrill, as I made my way into the district

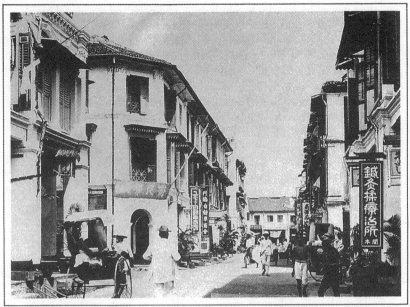

MALAY STREET

inhabited by the poorest Chinese. Somewhere in these narrow streets were houses where secret societies still held their meetings and where another set of laws and moral codes held sway. Somewhere in this teeming ant-heap of yellow humanity were the political agitators and the gang-robbers whose raids and hold-ups from time to time stirred a complacent European community to demand an increased vigilance from a police force which is both efficient and remarkably well-informed. But the illusion was only temporary. Malay Street itself brought me face to face with the new Singapore. Gone was Madame Blanche with her collection of Hungarians, Poles and Russian Jewesses – the frail army of white women recruited by the professional pimps from the poorest population of Central and Eastern Europe, and drifting farther East as their charms declined, *via* Bucarest, Athens and Cairo, until they reached the *ultima Thule* of their profession in Singapore.

There had been no English girls among them. On political grounds the British administration has always maintained a ban on the British prostitute. But here in the past, ship's officers of every nationality, and globe-trotters, travellers, miners and planters from up-country wasted

237

their money on an orgy to which drink and noise and occasional brawl-
ing supplied a discordant orchestra. Sometimes, a Malay princeling or
Chinese towkay would make his way discreetly to this sordid temple in
order to satisfy an exotic and perhaps politically perverted desire for the
embraces of the forbidden white women.

Gone, too, were the long rows of Japanese brothels with their lower
windows shuttered with bamboo poles behind which sat the waiting
odalisques, discreetly visible, magnificent in elaborate head-dress and
brightly coloured kimonos, heavily painted and powdered, essentially
doll-like and yet not without a certain charm which in romantic youths
like myself inspired a feeling more of pity than of desire. . . .

That drive through Malay Street will remain in my memory for longer
than the previous visits of my youth. Then one had been drunk and in
the company of others. And together we had taken possession of the
place. Or else one had driven down the street furtively, with the hood of
the rickisha up, afraid lest any pair of eyes behind the shuttered windows were witnesses to the white man's secret shame and not daring to
emerge until one had ascertained if Rose or Madeline or Wanda were
free.

Then there had been discreet and obsequious touts at the doors to
show the way and to carry messages. Now I felt no sense of self-
consciousness because the feeling of shame was absent. The street was
the same street. The houses, too, looked old, and must have been the
same houses that I had known a quarter-of-a-century before. But they
had been reconstructed. The ground floor was now a row of open
booths, where small shopkeepers plied their trade. The Europeans and
the Japanese had vanished. Like an army of ants the Chinese had taken
possession of the district, removing all vestiges of its former occupants.
In one booth a whole family of husband, wife, sons and daughters, were
ironing the day's washing. In another an old man, consumptive-looking
and almost hairless, was working an antiquated model of a sewing
machine. Around him, squatting Buddha-wise on the floor, were half a
dozen assistants patiently sewing buttons on to khaki suits. . . .

My last night in Singapore I kept to myself. It was to be devoted to a
return to the past. I should engage a rickisha puller, preferably one who
could speak no known language, and the rest of the evening would be
left to the whims of his mechanical jog-trot. Like a leaf before the wind I
should go wherever he chose to pull me.

I put my plan into effect after an excellent dinner. There had been a thunderstorm during the afternoon. But the skies had cleared, and under the starlit heavens there was a delicious coolness in the air. My rickisha puller was a scraggy, toothless old man. Like the harper in the *Lay of the Last Minstrel* he was admirably suited to perform the rites at the last rickisha ride that I shall ever take. For even if I ever return to the East, the rickisha will soon be a vehicle of the past.

I had some difficulty in clambering into my seat. Perhaps I had lost the knack. I had certainly added several stone to my weight since the days when a husky sweating giant used to pull me the long ten miles out to my estate at Pantai at ten cents a mile. Then I could sleep the whole way. But this was an uncomfortable ride. My puller spoke no Malay and no English. From his lips came a stream of unintelligible labials. I waved an arm towards the night. With a grin he seized the shafts, and off we jogged. Twenty-five years ago we should have pulled up at a brothel, for your rickisha puller, even if he is inarticulate, knows instinctively the tastes of the tourist, and in those days Malay Street was the obvious destination of a European setting out alone at night.

Fashions, however, have changed, and after a gentle trot my puller stopped before a gateway with a huge electric sign in English and flashing the words, "The New World". I got out and rather shyly followed the throng which was streaming through the open gates. Inside was a huge fair with theatres, opera, cinema, dancing-hall, side-shows, booths, refreshment stalls, and even a stadium. The crowd was of all classes and of all races. Naval ratings towered over squat Malays. If Chinese predominated, there was a fair sprinkling of Europeans and Eurasians. Tamils, Japanese, Arabs and Bengalis completed the racial conglomeration.

The noise was deafening. Next door to an open Chinese theatre with the usual accompaniment of gongs, a Malay operatic company was performing *Mashdur*. From the side-shows came an endless broadside of chatter and laughter. In the booths in the centre, Japanese and Chinese were selling toys which would have delighted the heart of any European child: voracious-looking dragons, clock-work crocodiles and snakes, miniature baby-carriages, wooden soldiers, and the quaintest of domestic animals.

Avoiding the cinema where alluring posters of Miss Mae West revealed the fact that *I'm No Angel* had been passed by the Singapore Board of Censors, I went into the dancing-hall. There was an excellent orchestra, hired, I think, from some liner. It was playing *Aufwiedersehen* when I came in, and a crowd of dancers, mostly young Chinese, the men in white European clothes with black patent-leather dancing shoes, the girls in their semi-European dresses slit at the side, filled the dancing-floor. Many of the dancers had their own partners. But when the dance was over I noticed a number of girls who left their partner as soon as the music stopped and went to join other girls in a kind of pen. They were the professional Chinese dancers who can be hired for a few cents a dance.

There were other Europeans dancing, and after asking an attendant how the thing was done I plucked up my courage and, as soon as the music started for the next dance, went over and engaged a partner. More intent on information than on pleasure I ambled slowly round the floor. I had no reason except my own clumsiness to feel self-conscious. My Chinese partner danced with the ethereal lightness of a Viennese. Her name was Tiger Lily, and she told me some of the secrets of her profession.

These Chinese girls are engaged by the management. They are very carefully selected, and breaches of discipline are severely punished. They are paid about eight cents a dance. Each dance is registered on a card, and at the end of the week the cards are vigilantly scrutinised. Girls who are in great request, and who can show a high average of dances, may be promoted. Others, whose engagements are below the fixed average, have their wages reduced. In the dancing-hall, at any rate, there is no social intercourse between guest and professional dancer. At the end of each dance the professional goes back to her barricaded seclusion. The decorum, indeed, was unimpeachable, and could not have been criticised even by a Wee Free minister in a North of Scotland parish. To me this model seemliness was even more extraordinary than the almost complete waiving of the colour bar in a British colony.

R.H. BRUCE LOCKHART
Return to Malaya (1936)

c. 1937

Yam Seng

British travel writer John MacCallum Scott and his wife spent a lazy month in Singapore, putting up at a boarding house. They then left for China, apparently undeterred by their discouraging encounter with Chinese food in Singapore.

Our boarding house in Singapore had once belonged to a Chinese millionaire in the great days of the rubber boom. It was a veritable palace with great spacious rooms and a fine central hall which did service as a dining-room. Our room opened directly off this hall, and was so large and lofty that the two beds, each draped in a mosquito net, looked like lonely ghosts hiding in a dark recess at one end of a drill-hall. The floor was tiled, and the furniture, though adequate, seemed dwarfed into insignificance by its surroundings. The adjoining bathroom was the essence of Spartan simplicity. Recent alterations had endowed it with a hand-basin and other offices, but there was no bath – only a shower sticking out from one of the walls, and a peculiarly Malayan institution known as a Shanghai jar, from which we ladled cold water over ourselves whenever we were tired of the monotony of the shower-bath.

The servants were all Chinese. Dressed in spotless white they padded about on bare feet all day long, attending to our every want, and reducing us to such a helpless pitch of dependency on them that, by the time our stay had come to an end, we had almost forgotten how to do anything for ourselves apart from dressing and eating. At any time of the day we had only to yell, "Boy", and he would be at our side in the twinkling of an eye. Everything from buying cigarettes to posting letters could be done from the depths of an arm-chair.

Our daily routine was deliciously lazy. At seven the Boy would bring early tea and a newspaper. Breakfast would be at half-past eight, and throughout the morning we would either read or write, or go into town

241

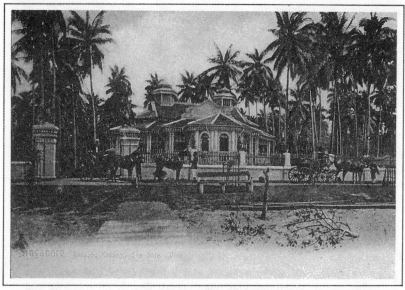

TANJONG KATONG SEA SIDE VILLA

to do some shopping, and have a gin sling at John Little's on the way.

Lunch would be at one, and afterwards we would crawl under our mosquito nets if the day was too oppressive to allow our staying awake any longer, or sit reading until tea time. After tea we would repair to the Swimming Club, and spend the remainder of the daylight alternating between swimming in the lukewarm water and sitting at the tables round its edge, drinking and gossiping with friends....

It was an idyllic existence, so completely divorced from all the actualities of life that we seemed to float through it as through a dream. Even now, over two years after, it requires only the faintest of hints – the mention of Singapore, the sight of a Malayan stamp on an envelope, or just laughter echoing over the water of a swimming pool – to bring it all back again, and set us longing for something that scarcely seems to belong to this world – the warm clasp of the tropics coupled with the freedom and ease which is the hall-mark of life as it is lived in Singapore....

Our first experience of Chinese food was not so pleasant ... The restaurant was on the roof, and so we travelled up to it in a very

242

modern lift together with some dozen Chinamen all decked out in spotless white ducks. When we reached it we found it practically full, and it was only with difficulty that we secured an empty table in a corner. At the time we did not realize that we were gatecrashing, but I do not think that our presence was resented . . .

At any rate, while we were still waiting for our dinner an old Chinese lady came across to us, and explained in pidgin English that a wedding reception was being held, that she was a very great friend of the bride's mother, and that the bride would be greatly honoured if the two ladies in our party would pay her a visit. The two ladies of our party were equally honoured, and were hustled away into a small room at the far end of the roof-garden, where they were introduced to the bride, a beautiful, fragile little thing, dressed in a lovely costume . . .

Meanwhile, the two of us who had been left behind were struggling with the menu and with the Chinese waiter who spoke no English and scarcely any Malay, and had at last succeeded in persuading him to bring us four portions of shark's fin soup. By the time Nora and her friend had returned it was waiting on the table. What a disappointment! It was a lukewarm gelatinous mess, which looked exactly like uncooked white of egg with shreds of what I suppose was shark's fin floating in it. We all stared at it despairingly, and each tried a mouthful. About a quarter of an hour later we persuaded the waiter to take the horrid thing away, and bring us instead a dish of what was described as mushrooms and prawns.

We passed the interval in watching the festivities. The guests were all men; again this was according to custom, for China is nothing if not a man's country, and on important occasions, such as a marriage, it is the men who feast, while the women remain demurely at home. At one end of the room a Chinese orchestra strummed away on an incredible variety of instruments, and produced a perfect bedlam of noise. Out in the street someone was honouring the occasion by letting off fire-crackers in a manner which seemed to bring Chicago dangerously near. A variety of foods covered the tables, and all the guests were making very merry. Anyone who maintains that the Chinese are impassive at all times ought to have been there to listen to the noise of laughter and shouting, and to watch the fatter, and therefore more virtuous, old gentlemen double themselves up on hearing a good story. Only the bride and bridegroom were missing, but they were due to appear shortly.

They arrived at the same time as our prawns and mushrooms, but the latter were so smothered in oil and fat that we could not make much of them, especially with chopsticks, and we were able to give our full attention to the ceremonies. . . .

Their manner of acting the host was different, however. They did not come together, but separately, the groom appearing first accompanied by his parents. In one hand he carried a bottle of brandy, and in the other a glass. At each table he stopped, and filled each guest's glass from the bottle. The guests at that table then rose to drink his health, which they did in a vigorous manner by emptying the whole glassful down their throats, turning it upside down at the end to show that not a drop was left, and some of them crying, "Yam seng", which is, I was told, the Chinese equivalent of "Bottoms up". The groom responded by taking a sip from his own glass, and then filled up the guests' glasses again before passing on to the next table. . . .

After he had visited about half the tables his bride appeared, escorted by her mother, and proceeded to make her round of the tables. Her progress, however, was more decorous, more in keeping with the humble position which women are supposed to occupy. Never once did she raise her eyes from the ground; not even as she served each of the guests with the ceremonial cup of tea, presenting it to them, according to custom with both hands; not even as she made her three ceremonial bows to each table. In return the guests never even looked at her, taking their téa exactly as though it had been handed to them by a waitress, and continuing their conversation as though the bride was not there. Presumably it was not good manners to look at her, for the Chinese are sticklers for etiquette.

When they had finished their rounds the bride and groom disappeared again, and the fun began to wax fast and furious as empty glasses were filled, and the cry, "Yam seng", was heard with ever-recurring frequency. Whether they were to come back or not we could not tell, as our lady interpreter had disappeared also. We waited for a little, but they still remained in seclusion, and as we were steadily getting hungrier and hungrier we made our way to the Swimming Club, where we regaled ourselves on good Christian ham sandwiches and beer.

JOHN H. MACCALLUM SCOTT
Eastern Journey (1939)

1939
Britain's Fortress

The English-language daily Singapore Herald, *a propaganda organ subsidised by the Japanese Government, first appeared in April 1939 – a few days before Tatsuki Fujii arrived in Singapore. As a journalist with American experience, Fujii came to work on the new paper.*

Singapore lay basking in the tropical sun when our ship sailed into the harbor on April 20, 1939. For hours that morning, I had stood on the deck waiting for the first glimpse of Singapore as the ship sailed serenely through blue waters between numerous green islands.

Finally, I caught a glimpse of the white buildings glinting in the sun. Singapore lay quietly asleep. How characteristic this was of Britain's fortress, I thought to myself.

Even before I disembarked, I was startled when the British Immigration Officer greeted me by name. It seemed that the police and even the newspaper reporters had been informed of my impending arrival.

Immediately upon landing, I was taken to the Police Station where I was questioned for more than an hour by Major Morgan, Chief of the Special Detective Branch. He asked me to give details of my trip from the United States, how long I had stayed in Japan and what I was going to do in Singapore.

Much to his disappointment, he learned very little from my replies. I told him that I had come to Singapore to work on the *Singapore Herald*. That was all I had to say. . . .

Singapore, on my arrival, was not a British city. It was predominantly Chinese with a good proportion of Indians, Malais and Arabs. The Japanese numbered only about 4,000. And yet the British ruled the destinies of the Asiatic population of 700,000 with selfish tyranny.

As in New Delhi, Hongkong and Shanghai, the British in Singapore had built imposing buildings in order to impress the masses. They had stationed troops in Malaya, not to fight, but to remind the Asiatics that the British ruled by virtue of force.

Bridges and roads were built not for public service, but solely for defense purposes. Schools were established in order that British history and language could be imposed upon the children. Hospitals and prisons were constructed because they were needed, not because of any humanitarian motive.

Wasn't it sufficient testimony of British oppression that the Supreme Court and the Changi Prison were the finest buildings in all of Malaya? . . .

In the early days of British colonial domination, some good men had been sent out in the Malayan Civil Service. Names like Sir Frank Swettenham and Sir Hugh Clifford stand out in Malayan history. They were sincerely interested in the welfare of the people and its culture. Sons of good families came out to Malaya, in those early days, as hardy pioneers in quest of adventure and fortune.

But as years went on, London grew lax and the social and economic misfits of the British Isles began to drift out to Malaya. There was nothing so obnoxious as a British colonial official. . . .

The poverty of the people increased the longer the British remained in Malaya. The slums of Singapore were world famous and in the midst of all this poverty and filth, the British lived in oblivious splendor.

Life in Singapore for the British was leisurely and comfortable. Most of them lived in the suburbs – Tanglin, Bukit Timah or along the East Coast – where it was cool. They built magnificent residences staffed with a retinue of Chinese and Malai servants.

Yes, Singapore was easy and comfortable for the middle-class English officials and businessmen. Many of the wives sprang from the petty bourgeoisie of England and Scotland. Many a police inspector had formerly walked the streets of London as a "bobbie" while more than one railway official had served his apprenticeship in an English dispatcher's office.

Scrubwomen, farmer's daughters and manicurists – all became Singapore "ladies." Many told amazing stories of aristocratic backgrounds which were refuted by the Cockney in their speech.

When Noel Coward, the celebrated English playwright and author, came out to Singapore, he was amazed at the smug, pretentious and bad manners of Singapore society.

After a visit to the Tanglin Club, one would-be lady asked him how he liked the Club.

246

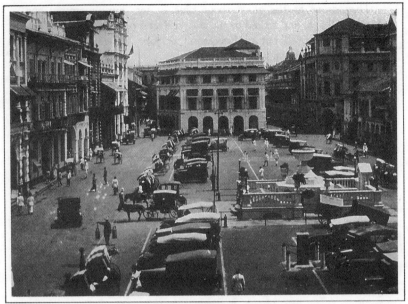

RAFFLES PLACE

"You know the Tanglin Club is one of our best clubs," the "lady" beamed.

Noel Coward turned to her and said, "After meeting your best people, now I know why there is such a shortage of servants in London."

Indeed, the British built up a life of superficial leisure in Singapore. While they drew handsome salaries and did no work, the efficient Chinese and Eurasian clerks slaved. It was only necessary for the British manager to make an appearance every day, sign the checks and dictate replies to letters that came from the head office in London.

The British rolled through town in limousines, lived in sumptuous villas and revelled at exclusive clubs while the rest of the Asiatic population starved, toiled, and died.

Even the young assistants lived well – usually in an apartment or a bachelors' mess which resembled a private club. All of the British managers and most of the younger assistants owned motor-cars driven by Malai chauffeurs. Their domestic needs were taken care of by a Malai or Chinese houseboy, Chinese cook, Malai gardener and a Chinese amah to do the laundry.

247

They drove to the office about nine or ten every morning, had lunch at 1 p.m. and retired to the club at 4 or 5 p.m. In the meantime, they often stepped out to Robinson's or John Little's for a cup of coffee or, more often, a gin bitter. . . .

For the younger bachelors, life in Singapore was very convenient. They usually started drinking at the Cricket Club, proceeded on to one of the three cabarets where they danced with a pretty Chinese or Eurasian partner and ended up at the cafes which lined Jalan Besar Road and Lavender Street. If the favors of certain dancers at the cabarets were unobtainable, they went along to one of the numerous brothels which served just as well.

And well after midnight, the trek from the clubs, the cabarets and cafes began – the British were going home to sleep. "It would be such a busy day tomorrow."

TATSUKI FUJII
Singapore Assignment (c. 1943)

1942

Heavy Casualties

Japanese air raids on Singapore started in December 1941 and continued into January. This account by A War Correspondent and headlined "Singapore Experiences its Worst Blitz" came just ten days before the Johore causeway was breached and the final siege of the island began.

Singapore suffered its worst blitz yesterday since the war began when two large waves of Japanese bombers flew over the city and dropped bombs on a residential district, causing little damage to property but fairly heavy casualties.

The bombs were dropped at random and the casualties were nearly all, if not all, among poor Asiatic civilians who had little to lose but their lives. The casualties are believed to have been about 50 dead and 150 injured.

I was one of many members of the Medical Auxiliary Service who turned out to assist in removing the casualties, and at the particular incident which I attended I saw a pathetic sight – dead, dying and injured.

But there was no murmuring among the injured and there was no panic among the civil population.

One of the patients, who was at death's door, that I attended said to me: "God will avenge this murder," as he was carried away on a stretcher to a waiting ambulance.

A good deal of the damage was done by blast from the bombs and some of the injuries were caused by broken glass and flying splinters, emphasising once again the desirability of shops on ground floors removing all glass from their windows. . . .

Some of the bombs fell on the hard road and concrete sidewalks and these appeared to create more blast than bombs which fell in soft ground. The craters were much smaller than those which I saw in some of the outlying districts on Saturday and Sunday, which suggests that in the town bigger blasts can be expected when bombs explode on hard surfaces.

At to-day's incidents there seemed to be a long delay between the time the bombs dropped and when assistance arrived, suggesting that there is still room for speeding up calls to the A.R.P. and M.A.S. control rooms and for energetic action by these controls when calls are received.

The raid was not without its amusing incidents one of which was when a taxi driver, not having heard the sirens, was driving along a main street when he heard bombs dropping. He left his taxi and sought shelter in a drain and within a few seconds the engine of his taxi was reposing near him in the drain having been completely torn from the chassis.

That there were not as many casualties as there might have been in yesterday's blitz was in a great measure due to people's taking cover when the bombers were overhead.

In one house the portico of which was blown down the inmates, numbering about 15, had taken to their shelter and escaped unhurt.

The Syce employed by these people owes his life to them. When the others went to the shelter he remained sitting in the car, which was parked under the portico. Two minutes before the portico was damaged he was ordered to take cover, and obeyed. The car was wrecked.

In another locality the only member of a household who was hurt when a bomb fell in the vicinity was the Tamil gardener. The master of this house, a European, is very insistent on all, including the servants, taking cover when a raid is on. In this instance the gardener, although called on to enter the shelter, stayed outside, and paid for his folly.

Business houses in the Singapore area affected by raids must be complimented for the promptness with which they resume service after their roof-spotters have given the "raiders passed" signal.

Yesterday, in one locality a shop was full of customers when the siren sounded. Business went on as usual until the roof-spotters gave the signal to take cover. With admirable calm, customers and staff proceeded to take cover. The rear portion of this building was hit, yet calm reigned, with the result that no one was injured.

A "casualty" occurred in the shop, however, soon after, when ammonia fumes escaped from some refrigerator coils caused rather a scare. One person, more nervous than the rest, tried to run away, stumbled and fell, and was hurt.

Within half an hour of the incident customers were being attended to again at this place.

At a restaurant, a wing of which had been damaged, customers were being served with tea and coffee. The morale of the servants and waiters had not been shaken in the least.

"Singapore Experiences its Worst Blitz"
The Straits Times, **January 21, 1942**

1942

Unconditional Surrender

Colonel Masanobu Tsuji was Chief of Operations & Planning Staff of the 25th Japanese Army. It was he who was responsible for the detailed planning of the Malayan campaign. The Japanese advanced six hundred miles through jungle country and after just seventy days of fighting captured Singapore on Sunday, 15 February.

After roughly a week of fighting since we crossed Johore Strait the ammunition accumulated for the assault on Singapore Island was nearly exhausted. We had barely a hundred rounds per gun left for our field guns, and less for our heavy guns. With this small ammunition supply it was impossible to keep down enemy fire by counter-battery operations.

Our only standby was Colonel Tanaka's 40-centimetre (16-inch) mortars. For mobility these were taken apart and loaded on handcarts, and at night placed in position in the front-line firing trench. Their shells, brought forward by the same means, thoroughly inspected and overhauled, were loaded and fired upon the enemy in Keppel Barracks at the rate of about one round every ten minutes.

The enemy were apparently resting while waiting for our attack. The Ito Battalion decided to launch an attack, and like men rising from their graves the men began to emerge from their trenches. Immediately a large number of British guns directed an intense barrage on the position. It seemed as if everyone on the battlefield would be suffocated by the dust and smoke from the bursting shells.

Takeda, the divisional chief of staff, who had come forward to direct the attack, came reluctantly to the conclusion that it was a sheer impossibility to proceed with it owing to the fact that the troops were exhausted by previous operations and the violent bombardment by the enemy. Arms and legs were flying through the air and heads scattered everywhere. Twisting my body like a crab and hiding my head behind an old tree I wished to myself that I had a steel helmet. A soldier, edging close to me, took off his own and put it on my head. We were complete strangers to each other. "Mr Staff Officer," he said, "it is dangerous to be without a steel helmet. Please wear this one." I thanked him and returned it to him, but he did not put it on his head again. I was deeply moved by the spirit of self-sacrifice of this soldier with whom I had not even a nodding acquaintance.

The regimental headquarters trench became shallower every time a shell exploded close to it. Frequently we were half buried. At last, carrying the regimental colours, we moved out of the trench and sought shelter behind the brick wall of a wrecked house, to which we clung like geckos. A soldier beside me had his head blown off, and blood was scattered everywhere. Two of his comrades stood up holding a blanket. "How will this do for a coffin?" asked one. They wrapped the corpse in the blanket and carried it on their shoulders to an abandoned trench about twenty yards in the rear. The regimental adjutant called to them, "It's too dangerous to bury him now. You'll be wiped out by a shell. Do it later." Undeterred, the two men carried on with their self-appointed task. Several times they were enveloped in the smoke and dust of bursting shells and we thought they had been killed, but after the smoke of each explosion cleared away they were to be seen still digging. It was an act of madness. . . .

The furious bombardment eased off about four o'clock in the afternoon and moved away from the Ito Battalion. I started homewards thinking, "If the enemy resists in this manner he probably contemplates fighting from house to house and it will take more time to capture the fortress. Our artillery ammunition is almost exhausted. We will have to concentrate on a new plan." Tired and heavy-footed, my orderly and I moved back along the road by which we had come that morning. . . .

As the day was gradually drawing to a close, I sorrowfully said farewell to Staff Officer Hashimoto, who was leaving Headquarters. I began to walk down the hill when I was called to answer an excited call on the telephone. Putting the receiver to my ear I said, "What is the matter? Is it urgent at this time of day?" Trembling with excitement the voice of my dear friend Staff Officer Hayashi answered, "The enemy has surrendered! Has surrendered!"

Unconsciously dropping the receiver I thought, "Ah! Seventy days of fighting . . . Keppel Barracks and the death struggle . . . Jitra's bloody battle." Like a magic lantern it all flashed before my mind. How would the heart of the nation be when this news came over the radio? It seemed a dream. Only a few moments ago we were engaged in a life-and-death struggle. "Perhaps I am dreaming," I thought. I pinched the flesh of my thigh hard through my trousers. I was certainly awake and in my right senses. It was no dream. From several places in the firing line cheering voices rose in the air. Then, originating in some corner, the Japanese National Anthem, *Kimi Ga Yo*, spread in a wave over the battlefields.

During the day on the 5th Division front the battle had raged as violently as in the Keppel Barracks area. Our front line had only been able to advance to the southern end of the reservoir. The troops had never before been under such heavy shellfire, from which the front-line trenches afforded very little shelter. The division had attacked from the main-road sector supported by the full strength of the "Tiger's Cub" Tank Brigade, but the troops were finally brought to a standstill at half-past three in the afternoon. Then suddenly, ahead of the front line which was renewing its assault along the central highway, there appeared a large white flag.

Major Wylde, an English staff officer, came bearing the flag of truce. Like lightning this was reported to Bukit Timah headquarters. Immediately on receiving the news Staff Officer Sugita, in charge of intelligence, who was in a plaster cast because of a broken collar-bone, was taken by car to the front line, where he personally delivered to the bearer of the flag of truce documents which had been prepared in anticipation at our Army Headquarters. The British staff officer at once returned to Singapore with them to enable the British commander of the fortress to consider our proposals . . .

The streamlined motor car with the Union Jack and the white flag crossing each other stopped in front of the Ford Car factory north of the three-pronged Bukit Timah road. The British Commander, Lieutenant-General Percival, accompanied by Brigadier Torrens, Brigadier Newbigging (Deputy Adjutant-General) and Major Wylde, were led to the place of interview by Staff Officer Sugita. General Yamashita, who was roughly five minutes behind time, entered followed by his staff officers, exchanged handshakes, and took his seat. How did the English general feel surrendering to his enemy after defeat? The faces of the four English officers were pale and their eyes bloodshot. General Yamashita indicated to General Percival a document written in English, saying, "I wish you to answer these questions very briefly."

The questions and answers were:

"Does the British Army surrender unconditionally?" – "Yes."

"Are there any Japanese prisoners of war?" – "Not even one man."

"Are there any Japanese men held prisoner?" – "All Japanese civilian prisoners have been sent to India. The guarantee of their position is being entrusted to the Government of that country."

"Do you agree to this document unconditionally?" – "Please wait until tomorrow morning for the answer."

"Then, in that case, up till tomorrow morning we will continue the attack. Is that all right, or do you consent immediately to unconditional surrender?" – "Yes."

"Well, then, there will be a cessation of hostilities from 10 p.m. Japanese time. The British Army, using a thousand men as a police force, will please maintain order. In case of any violation of these terms a full-scale attack on Singapore will immediately commence."

General Percival then said, "I wish to receive a guarantee of the safety of the lives of the English and Australians who remain in the city."

"You may be sure of that. Please rest assured. I shall positively guarantee it."

In this way the curtain dropped on the campaign for the occupation of Singapore.

COL. MASANOBU TSUJI
Singapore: The Japanese Version **(1952)**
Trans. Margaret E. Lake (1960)

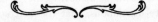

1942

Escape

When the surrender came, many who had fought for Singapore decided to leave – if they could – rather than face imprisonment. Lieutenant-General Gordon Bennett, Commander of the Australian Imperial Forces in Malaya, was one of those who escaped to tell their story, although he was later to face official censure for abandoning his command.

Everyone was stunned by the decision to surrender. All knew for many days that there was no other alternative. Nevertheless the end came as a shock. Their war was over. Their hopes and ambitions were shattered. They were to become prisoners of the despised Japanese. They were to submit to the ignominious position of spending the rest of the war behind barbed wire – at the mercy of the Japanese, who had a very bad reputation for the way in which they treated their prisoners. Their wives and children, their parents, their friends, their homes in Australia were suddenly cut off. None knew when they would see them again. Proud men accept such servility with bad grace.

During the last few days, many decided to endeavour to escape. I discussed with senior officers the idea of urging the men to do so, telling them the best means of achieving the objective. All gave their opinions, which were unanimous, that the outcome was so hazardous that it would be attended with heavy casualties. It was left to the men themselves to act as they thought best. A number of the staff had banded themselves into escape groups. They had equipped themselves for the journey and had made their plans.

I, personally, had made this decision some time previously, having decided that I would not fall into Japanese hands. My decision was fortified by the resolve that I must at all costs return to Australia to tell our people the story of our conflict with the Japanese, to warn

256

them of the danger to Australia, and to advise them of the best means
of defeating the Japanese tactics.

My aide-de-camp, Lieutenant Gordon Walker, had mentioned my
resolve to Major Charles Moses. Between them they undertook the
self-imposed task of getting me back to our beloved Australia. We
three formed a pact to escape together and we decided that if any of
the three should be wounded or captured during the attempt, the
others were to continue, leaving the unfortunate one rather than
jeopardize the escape of the rest.

Brigadier Callaghan was my next senior officer. He was weak from
a recent attack of malaria. I went to his shelter and told him of my
resolve, asking him to let the Japanese think I had escaped some days
earlier, should they ask any questions as to my whereabouts. When
I called I found him seated in a room, badly lighted by a kerosene
lamp. He seemed dazed. He was an old friend and a very good soldier.
Our farewell was short but full of deep feeling. I then said good-bye
to the rest of my staff: Jim Thyer, my G.S.O.I., Bill Kent Hughes, my
A.Q., Brigadier Maxwell, Colonel Derham, and the others. All knew
of my determination.

Returning to my quarters, I hurriedly went through my belongings,
selecting the minimum needs for the journey, on the assumption that
I would have a jungle tramp for 150 to 200 miles to Malacca or Port
Dickson.

I found that Major Moses had returned with my car and his new-
found Chinese friend. With Gordon Walker, we drove off on our
adventure, he being at the wheel of my car.

Our headquarters were less than two miles from the enemy troops
and our journey took us through the black and silent city of Singapore,
which we anticipated would, even at that time, be occupied by Japanese
soldiers. The city smelt of burnt timber, explosives and – blood. The
streets were filled with rubble from the bomb-torn pavements, with
overturned cars and trams, wires from the electric light and telephone
service lying loosely about the streets. We were making for the coast
near the Kalang aerodrome. On the way we were bailed up at the
point of the bayonet by some stray men of the Gordon Highlanders
who demanded to know if it were a fact that the war was over. On
being told "yes" they quickly vanished. Pushing onward, nearly wrecking
the car in the bomb craters on the road, we arrived at Beach Road
and turned down a dark lane leading to the sea-front. The place was

silent as the grave. This district, in normal times, was a seething mass of humanity, brightened by the multi-coloured garments hanging on poles from the upstairs windows of this thickly populated area. Now everyone had gone. The previous day the buildings had been burnt out by Japanese incendiary bombs.

Our Chinaman alighted to search for his friend from whom we were buying our boat. The friend had gone and his boat was missing. Our guide piloted us towards the water-front but was stopped by a guard of an Indian unit, not yet aware that hostilities had ceased. I stayed by the car, feeling very lonely but not afraid, although the atmosphere was eerie, while the rest of the party went forward in search of the officer of the guard. This officer piloted us past his sentries to the water-front. We moved through the village silently, hugging the buildings closely, as two Japanese officers had just arrived in the vicinity. He then said good-bye, shaking us warmly by the hand and wishing us good luck. He wished he could accompany us.

Reaching the water's edge, we were picking our way along a rough track when we were stopped by another guard. We managed to talk our way past it, arriving at a jetty where we expected to find a small boat. It was gone. The dark night was dimly lighted by the glow from a burning petrol dump on a nearby island. All was silent, save for the gentle lapping of the water against the stone sea-wall. Our Chinese guide left us, refusing any payment for his trouble, so I gave him my car which we had left in the village.

Seeing some sampans fifty yards or so from the shore we decided to take one. Gordon Walker stripped off his uniform, dived into the highly phosphorescent sea and swam out to the boats, which he found were securely lashed. With some difficulty he cut the lashing of the first one, then another and then a third before he could find one that he could handle. This he brought to the shore, showing clearly that he was a sheep farmer rather than a boatman. We quickly tossed in our belongings and clambered down the piers of the jetty, anxious to get under way. As we were pulling away, a party of men rushed wildly on to the jetty, gesticulating and calling excitedly for us to return. At first we feared they were Japanese but their language soon showed them to be friends. They were eight British planters serving in the Malay Volunteer Forces. We took them aboard and set off once again for our unknown destination, struggling slowly with our overcrowded craft through the hundreds of sampans that choke the sea in all Eastern ports. The boat kept slewing round, the oarsmen being rather unused to sampans. We fouled boat after boat as we passed through the hundreds of sampans that were lying off shore. Soon the tempers of everyone became frayed. There was plenty of cursing and complaining; we were making little progress. I visualized failure and pictured an early return to land, and an attempt to escape via the mainland in accordance with our original plans. Moses suggested that we should row round to Jurong River – a mere ten miles – where we could go ashore behind the Japanese lines and make our way north on foot. One of the planters then said that he had been told that day by a Harbour Trust official that it may be possible to obtain a *tongkan* to transport him to Sumatra. As if some guardian angel were helping us, suddenly out of the darkness loomed a large black object which turned out to be a *tongkan*. We had realized that the small boat was an impossible means of getting across to Sumatra and quickly climbed on board the *tongkan*. We kicked the clumsy sampan away with finality and set it drifting towards the shore. On board we found two men, very wet and ill. They had swum out from the shore, their escape being marred by the loss of two of their party who were drowned, as they could not make the distance. We found the Chinese owner of our new-found craft busy with his opium pipe. He had a crew of two. He refused to take us to our goal, Sumatra, saying he wanted more opium and could get it only at Singapore. While one of the planters was haggling in Chinese, I investigated the craft and found it full of A.A. ammunition which we discovered had been brought from Seletar on the north side of the island to Singapore. This ammunition was stored in metal boxes and thrown into the hold in a very haphazard way and covered with a tarpaulin. It was level as a newly ploughed field and as hard as flint. But it was a safe refuge and – well, we were not prisoners of the Japanese. The haggling with the owner continued, so we held a conference and decided to take charge of his *tongkan* and put to sea. We found an American, a gunner in the Hong Kong and Singapore A.A. Artillery who said he could manage the boat. Seeing that we were desperate and determined, the Chinese owner agreed to take us to Sumatra for an unnamed sum of money. Moses gave him 150 Straits dollars on account and promised him more when we reached our destination. Finally at 0100 hours on 16 February the opium pipe was put aside, the sail set, the anchor raised and we commenced our journey.

Our first problem was to take our boat, so heavily laden with explosives, through the mine-fields defending Singapore. We just shut our eyes and sailed straight ahead. By some miraculous turn of Fortune's wheel we hit nothing and passed on our way, some of our party already deep in an exhausted sleep.

We found that there were nineteen of us on board (excluding the crew), a few more escapees arriving just before we left.

We crawled into the hold which was covered with a tarred tarpaulin resting on bamboo poles. Two planters were appointed as food controllers and all food and water was handed to them, those who swam out being unable to make any contribution. We decided to ration the food and water so that it would last four days, the time we estimated the trip to Sumatra would take.

I peered out into the night and saw the moon rising over the island. We passed near the island of Blakang Mati, which was occupied by the enemy and went to the south of Palau Bukum, on which a large oil tank was burning fiercely. We felt relieved. We were leaving Singapore and the Japanese.

LIEUT-GEN. H. GORDON BENNETT
Why Singapore Fell (1945)

Tale-end

The following pieces, specially selected for this new
edition, begin once again in the years of the nineteenth
century and take the reader through to the time of the
Pacific War. They throw an intriguing light into yet more
corners of Singapore's past.

1858

A Valuable Introduction

_____

Albert Smith stopped briefly in Singapore en route to China. He wanted to discover all he could about the Chinese, in preparation for an exhibition, "Mr. Albert Smith's China", which he was to put on in London the following year. Whampoa, who had come to Singapore as a teenager in 1830 to help with his father's business, was far from being a typical immigrant.

Saturday, 14th. [August] – Land in sight from the time of getting up. Dropped anchor in Singapore roads at 10.30, and on shore with one of the passengers getting a large bedroom between us, at the Hotel de l'Esperance, on the Esplanade, at Singapore. Went, first of all, to Captain Marshall, the P. and O. agent, who was very polite, and told me I must know Mr. Whampoa – a leading China merchant, living close by. He sent me round, with a clerk, and a very valuable introduction it proved to me. I found Whampoa – as he is universally called – sitting at his warehouse door, watching his boat unlading. He spoke English perfectly, and received me with excellent English courtesy. After a little talk he dispatched me, with one of his men, to see the Buddhist Temples, or Joss Houses, in the town. They are very striking to a stranger, and elaborate in hideous images, gold, and carving. A man was in one, burning joss-stick, and throwing up two bits of wood, to tell his fortune from the manner in which they fell. Grim figures every where met the eye; and there were two large tanks, without water, at the bottom of which a few sacred tortoises crawled lazily about. At the gate was the statue of a lion, with a large ball carved in his mouth, which turned round but would not come out. When we had been over the temple, on which was hung an enormous drum and bell – to call the Joss's attention, when they think he is not listening – the priest took a bottle of stout from behind an altar, which I enjoyed very much. I gave him a rupee, and the old boy "chin-

chin'd" me to the ground. I saw many other temples, but none so grand as this. Back to Whampoa, who asked me to dine with him that day. I then took my umbrella, and wandered about the town, infinitely amused and interested. The shops are all under porticos, and the houses only a story high – all kept and inhabited by Chinese. Their names and trades were mostly painted in vermilion, and sometimes gilt, on black boards, and written perpendicularly. Tailors and barbers are very frequently combined, in the same shop. The tailors sat at tables covered with fine matting, and the barbers' strops were very long and hung from the ceiling. They shaved without lather, but with rice-water, and then shampoo'd their customers, and with many little instruments cleaned their eyes and ears. Scribes sat gravely at tables under the porticos. One was doing a book. It was on very thin paper, and under this he placed a guide, so that the characters showed through. These he traced, working very quickly. Another was a grey-headed old man, like an owl, with a white beard and whiskers, and wearing enormous pantomime spectacles. He was adding vermilion dots and rings, here and there, to the pages already done. Over the doorways fluttered little labels of red paper, gilt and perforated, put there on New Year's day. In the carpenters' shops the planes had a handle on each side; and one man was doing some work, and at the same time rolling a grindstone backwards and forwards with his feet over some blue powder in a concave trough. In front of some of the houses were curious representations of birds, animals, and flowers, made of broken pottery, let into the cement. I also saw a walking *restaurateur*. His "establishment" consisted of two square stands, with little rails three parts round the top. In one was a fire-place, and small copper, with a store of fuel underneath. On the top of the other, in little bowls, were his chief articles of food – oysters, picked shrimps, onions, a sort of maccaroni, and scraps of meat and duck. Underneath these were drawers with more things in them. While there, a customer ate a little basin of soup with oysters in it, with a horn spoon. It all looked very clean, and appeared an excellent thing. When no customer came the man knocked two bits of bamboo together, to attract attention.

At half-past four I went back to Whampoa, and sat and talked with him at the door, whilst the people came up offering ducks and poultry for sale, as well as canes and walking-sticks. In the street they sold bits of sugar cane, about nine inches long, to the boys, with slices of pine-apple, for the smallest possible coin. Paid a visit to Mr. Woods, of the *Straits Times* – an important paper out here. His compositors were all foreigners, and he showed me his different presses, chiefly American. One small hand one, by Orcutt, of Boston, was one of the cleverest things I ever saw for simple rapidity. Captain Maguire now joined me, and we went off to Whampoa's in his carriage.

. . . The house, here, was superbly furnished in the English style, but with lanterns all about it. At six the guests arrived – mostly English – including Captain Marshall, and all dressed in short white jackets and trousers. The dinner was admirably served, in good London style, and all the appointments as regards plate, glass, wines, and dishes, perfect. The quiet, attentive waiting of the little China boys deserved all praise. After dinner, we lounged through the rooms, decorated with English prints of the Royal family, statuettes, *"curios"* from every part of the world, and rare objects in jade-stone, and crackle china, also a portrait of our host's son, who is being educated in Edinburgh. He was in English dress.

About nine we all drove down, in various traps, to the theatre. It was an enormous tent, as big as the old Free Trade Hall, at Manchester; and made entirely of bamboos and matting . . . There was a large Chinese scroll at the back, on which was the name of the theatre. The female characters were played by men, who all sang in a shrill *falsetto*, and the plot was very straggling and obscure. The change of scene was effected by merely taking a chair away, or putting on a screen; and when the musicians were not playing, they had a pipe. . . . At last Whampoa said, "Now they are married, and it's all over", so we left, and he drove me to the hotel. The people had all gone to bed, but I kicked up a native who was lying asleep on the ground before the porch, and he lighted me to my room. The other passenger was already in his bed; and I soon got into mine and fell asleep, very tired. I was not troubled with the mosquitoes, although I did not let down the curtains.

Sunday, 15th. – To breakfast with Captain Marshall, at his bungalow. Passed a burial ground at the side of the hill, with many Chinese tombs; also several hovels, where they sold bits of pine-apple, plantains, and dried fish; and houses built on piles, in the low-water mud. Noticed a dram-shop, with a sign "Paddy-Goose, by Madras Bob". Captain Marshall's bungalow is charmingly situated on a hill, overlooking the magnificent harbour and docks, now being built by the Peninsular and Oriental Company. We had some of the best mutton I have tasted out; and a prawn curry was – for curry – a great success. The prawns were as large as cray-fish. To the hotel for lunch; and several of us had some champagne, to drink the health of Mr. Purves, whom we left here. Had a good row about the bill. I have a great affection for hotels generally, and this formed no exception. They wanted to charge me three dollars (12s.6d.) for my bed and the half of the room. The proprietress, Madame Esperanza, had been, as some said, a baroness; according to others, a lady's maid. We, however, made her take off two-thirds of the bill. On board the *Norna*, at 2 P.M., and started at once. In the night, the cockroaches, or rats, or both, finished the hind part of one of my shoes, and carried one of my slippers clean away.

ALBERT SMITH
***To China and Back* (1859)**

Glossary
Chin-Chin – a corruption of the Chinese salutation *Ch'ing Ch'ing*, which answers to our good-bye, presents compliments, etc.
Esplanade – original name of the grassy area now known as the Padang.

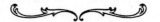

1889

We Our Noble Selves

When Rudyard Kipling visited Singapore he was leaving India, the country of his birth, and moving to England where, at the age of 24, he became an immediate success as a writer. On seeing how far the Chinese were already managing affairs in Singapore, Kipling remarked drily: "England is by the uninformed supposed to own the island."

When one comes to a new station the first thing to do is to call on the inhabitants. This duty I had neglected, preferring to consort with Chinese till the Sabbath, when I learnt that Singapur went to the Botanical Gardens and listened to secular music.

All the Englishmen in the island congregated there. The Botanical Gardens would have been lovely at Kew, but here, where one knew that they were the only place of recreation open to the inhabitants, they were not pleasant. All the plants of all the tropics grew there together, and the orchid-house was roofed with thin battens of wood – just enough to keep off the direct rays of the sun. It held waxy-white splendours from Manila, the Philippines, and tropical Africa – plants that were half-slugs, drawing nourishment apparently from their own wooden labels; but there was no difference between the temperature of the orchid-house and the open air; both were heavy, dank, and steaming. I would have given a month's pay – but I have no month's pay! – for a clear breath of stifling hot wind from the sands of Sirsa, for the darkness of a Punjab dust-storm, in exchange for the perspiring plants, and the tree-fern that sweated audibly.

Just when I was most impressed with my measureless distance from India, my carriage advanced to the sound of slow music, and I found myself in the middle of an Indian station – not quite as big as Allahabad, and infinitely prettier than Lucknow. It overlooked the gardens that sloped in ridge and hollow below; and the barracks were set in much greenery, and there was a mess-house that suggested long and cooling drinks, and there walked round about a British band. It was just We Our Noble Selves. In the centre was the pretty Memsahib with light hair and fascinating manners, and the plump little Memsahib that talks to everybody and is in everybody's confidence, and the spinster fresh from home, and the bean-fed, well-groomed subaltern with the light coat and fox-terrier. On the benches sat the fat colonel, and the large judge, and the engineer's wife, and the merchant-man and his family after their kind – male and female met I them, and but for the little fact that they were entire strangers to me, I would have saluted them all as old friends. I knew what they were talking about, could see them taking stock of one another's dresses out of the corners of their eyes, could see the young men backing and filling across the ground in order to walk with the young maidens, and could hear the 'Do you think so's' and 'Not really's' of our polite conversation. It is an awful thing to sit in a hired carriage and watch one's own people, and know that though you know their life, you have neither part nor lot in it.

I am a shadow now; alas! alas!
Upon the skirts of human nature dwelling,

I said mournfully to the Professor. He was looking at Mrs. ——, or some one so like her that it came to the same thing. 'Am I travelling round the world to discover *these* people?' said he. 'I've seen 'em all before. There's Captain Such-an-one and Colonel Such-another and Miss What's-its-name as large as life and twice as pale.'

The Professor had hit it. That was the difference. People in Singapur are dead-white – as white as Naaman – and the veins on the backs of their hands are painted in indigo.

It is as though the Rains were just over, and none of the womenfolk had been allowed to go to the hills. Yet no one talks about the unhealthiness of Singapur. A man lives well and happily until he begins to feel unwell. Then he feels worse because the climate allows him no chance of pulling himself together – and then he dies. Typhoid fever appears to be one gate of death, as it is in India; also liver. . . .

Nobody would speak to me in the gardens, though I felt that they ought to have invited me to drink, and I crept back to my hotel to eat six different fresh chutnies with one curry.

RUDYARD KIPLING
From Sea to Sea (1900)

1902

Local Colour

Sir Richard Winstedt's memoirs, discovered and published only after his death, contain this account of a very full day spent in Singapore on his first arrival in the country. Then just a 24-year-old Cadet, he was later to become Director of Education for the Straits Settlements and the Federated Malay States.

I was met at the quay by two fellow cadets, a few years senior to myself in the service, who carried me off to the Singapore Club for lunch. It was the old two-storeyed Club then, not the Club of today that reminds one of a mis-shapen snack bar in a great soulless railway-station. There was the old shabby intimate Club and along the sea-front there were the old plastered offices wooden-verandahed of the type that faced every anchorage from Port Said to Hongkong. The view from the Club verandah must have been as colourful as a Bonnard then, as I was to find it in after years, but I could not see much of it that day on account of what looked like a row of billowy white bedding stretched on chairs between me and the verandah: inspection revealed it to be a line of duck-clad period paunches, belonging to Gargantuan members, who reclined almost horizontally in Burma chairs apparently awaiting the Last Trump. My host talked mostly of polo, an exotic sport in Malaya, and I discovered that he was a keen gardener and a confirmed bachelor with a dislike of Honolulu Creeper because it reminded him of Eurasian weddings. His companion informed me that he was in the Secretariat and had a great future, as he was adept at drafting dispatches which the Colonial Office could read in either of two ways. Years afterwards he was to retire from the service prematurely because on one important occasion his hand lost its cunning and he made a rash unequivocal statement.

At this distance of time the Singapore of 1902 is little more to me than a labyrinth of beautiful laterite roads, colour-washed two-

270

storeyed shop-houses, flame-of-the-forest trees and a Gothic Cathedral that might have been a chapter by Walpole inserted in a novel by Conrad. In a gharry, that was as clumsy as a sedan-chair copied by a village carpenter, we drove into what was then the courtyard and later the lounge of the Hotel de l'Europe. At that prehistoric period we walked along a wooden verandah to our bedrooms and bathed out of Shanghai jars. Before dinner a fellow cadet and I visited the bar and seeing a list of cocktails ordered a Manhattan, but the Chinese boy shook his head: we pointed to the second, the third, the fourth mixture on that list, only to see his face grow more smilingly bland and the shake of his head as emphatic as Chinese etiquette and a pigtail would allow. At last an English-speaking attendant told us that the list dated back to the day of an American barman, who had sailed away to Shanghai. Nowadays every Chinese house-boy in Malaya can shake a Manhattan and a Martini, but in those days his master had to be content with sherry or a *pahit*, namely gin (or whisky) and bitters, with water to taste. . . .

Entering the Europe's dining-room I saw in the middle aisle the biggest brass bowl I have ever encountered, a Burmese vessel as large as a font and adorned with Buddhas seated in a maze [of] stylised foliation. It is the bit of local colour I recollect most vividly in the Singapore of 1902, and now that the Hotel de l'Europe has been killed by the great slump and its site acquired for a new Supreme Court, I am glad to know the great brass bowl was bought to adorn the lounge of Raffles Hotel. To many it is far more than a curio; for in its cavernous depth lives the genie of a hotel that before its eclipse was for years the scene of Singapore's European revelry by night, a genie that, nourished in 1902 on the humble smell of red Macassar fish, Bombay butter and salted Calcutta hump, came after the war to revel in the more delicate odour of chicken Lucullus, Homard à l'Américaine and Punch Romain.

After dinner we went to a music-hall called the Tingle-Tangle, where an old European livid with drink titubated out of the door as we entered to order a *kunchi* beer and listen to a chorus of fat white Austrian girls, dressed in the scarlet and green and white of the Tyrol and looking as if they would like to yodel, if the dank heat would not turn that exercise into a gargle. At the Tingle-Tangle we picked up a young subaltern stiff as a ramrod and speaking in the staccato barrack-room tones of the British officer of the stage. Having landed two days earlier than ourselves he offered to show us life and took us in

271

smooth rickshaws to a house with green shutters in the then famous Malay Street, where like orchids in a conservatory Japanese ladies sat behind bamboo-bars with paper flower-gardens on their heads, too utterly doll-like to excite desire: Will Rogers in a Rotary Club speech remarked that in that immoral cesspool Singapore he found nothing wilder than a Dutch wife, but that generous bolster is suggestive beside the chaste porcelain pillow of a Geisha. We drank more horribly warm beer and we talked pidgin English and then, bred in an age and class of inhibitions, returned to our hotel. . . .

At noon, wilting and damp in English flannels, we were glad to board a B.I. steamer for Penang.

SIR RICHARD WINSTEDT
Start from Alif: Count from One (1969)

Glossary
Tingle-Tangle – a concert and dance hall in North Bridge Road; from at least the 1890s.

1911

The Ship

As a youngster Clive Dalton came to live on Pulau Brani overlooking Keppel Harbour in "a fine spacious bungalow high up on a hill". His father was in the British army, but many of Clive's new friends were local Malay boys.

The Malays used to make wonderful model *sampans*, which I desired above all things in the world; and several of my friends had promised me one. But the Malay has an incurable habit of procrastination, and I never got my *sampan* because it was always put off until to-morrow.

There came a time, however, when I secured a prize even greater than a *sampan*, and that was a ship of strange design which I found upon the beach at Blakang Mati. It was of a kind I had seen the Pulau Brani islanders making, and I knew it had great religious significance. Periodically there was some kind of religious festival on the island, and then these ships were made, blessed, and sent out to sea, laden with fruits and spices and all manner of foodstuffs as an offering to the gods. They were beautifully made and unlike any craft I had ever seen, with two decks and a high poop, and they were manned by little wooden sailors and armed with wooden cannon. I imagine that they were reproductions of the pirate vessels of old. The food was made up in little packages and stowed in the hold, and the ship was launched with much ceremony and the burning of incense.

I had on occasion seen these ships at sea and had begged *sampan*-wallahs and canoe-men to take me out to them, but none would ever go near them. These ships were sacred.

And then one day I found one on the beach at Blakang Mati: a magnificent specimen, four feet long and a foot wide, and in perfect condition. . . .

When Ali saw me he gave a shout and his eyes grew wide with horror. . . . He told me of the awful things that happened to people

273

who took the ships that were meant for the gods. He begged me to put her back in the sea, and all would be well. He would himself burn incense and offer prayers on my behalf.

It was all useless. That ship was the find of a life-time and nothing would induce me to give her up.

Jaafar was even more upset when he heard and refused to play with the ship. He, too, entreated me to send her out to sea, but I refused and relations were strained. I had to go and play by myself with the ship, and for the first time I was completely out of harmony with my Malay friends.

Silly superstitions!

I had a lovely time that evening with my new ship, and I only hoped that when I went to school in the morning and told Ali that there had been no ghosts, he would stop being so silly about it. . . .

I turned and tucked the mosquito-net about me and prepared myself for sleep. Ali's threat of ghosts could not keep me awake and I was soon deep in dreams. . . .

And then I passed through a green twilight where everything was vague and ominous and fear haunted my footsteps and sinister things stirred in the shadows, until I came to a sea that glowed with an unearthly green light, and there was my ship, grown to full size and manned by a ruffianly looking crew . . .

. . . I passed into a deeper darkness from which I emerged from time to time to find myself still on the deck of this awful ship. There were times when I seemed to leave the ship and float in the air above her, and then I saw her sailing swiftly across the dark waters of that strange sea; and even then I could see myself aboard. . . .

There were times, too, when I had fleeting moments of consciousness, when I saw again the square of light that was the window I knew, and the anxious faces of my relatives bending over me; and once I came right out of my body and saw myself lying there under the mosquito-net, with my face white and my eyes sunk deep in my head. But even then I still saw that ship, and I always came back to her.

How long it lasted I do not know. For days I hovered on the brink of death. The doctors were baffled and were unable to say whether I should live or die. I knew more than they. I knew that if I could bring myself back to tell them what to do, I should get well. I knew. That was why I struggled. I tried to get to them to tell them to take that ship and launch her on the sea, but I could not reach them. That ship was still on the veranda where I had left her on the day I found her. If I could reach the veranda . . . I tried to. Even while in the throes of delirium I tried to get out of bed, but they held me back, not knowing what was in my mind.

In the morning I was weak but normal. I was back in my own room, and I smiled at the R.A.M.C. doctor who came to see me.

"I think he could sit out on the veranda," said the doctor. "It will do him good."

They took me out on to the veranda and I looked for the ship. It was not where I had left it. I asked my mother about it. She said it was where I had left it, and was amazed to see that it was gone.

I knew then what had happened. . . .

It was as I thought. They had known; and they had saved me. What unknown influences had been at work, I could not even guess, but I knew that from the depths of subconsciousness where I lay, I had reached out to Jaafar, and Jaafar, understanding those things better than the white people, had responded. It was he who had stolen the ship and launched her upon the sea. He never admitted it, but I knew.

CLIVE DALTON
A Child in the Sun (1937)

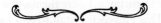

1927

Smuggling Opium

The smoking of opium (chandu) was permitted in Singapore until the early '40s, but its supply was a government monopoly – and a substantial revenue-earner. However, as 29-year-old Andrew Gilmour of the Malayan Civil Service (M.C.S.) found, there were people inside and outside the Department who preferred to trade on their own account.

One of the most interesting and exciting periods of my life came when I was unexpectedly seconded to a post outside the M.C.S. Cadre altogether in June 1927. . . .

It came about like this. A brilliant ex-"Mountie", who . . . was attached to the Detective Branch in Singapore, made a secret report alleging that several members of the staff of the Preventive Service of the Government Monopolies Department (the predecessor of the Customs and Excise Department) were themselves actively engaged in smuggling opium. This Preventive Staff were a locally recruited very mixed bag, including ex-police inspectors and prison warders.

. . . It was decided to ask the Police to second a very senior man to take over the Preventive Service and I undertook to act temporarily until one was available. This interim period lasted for 5 months, during which I lived in a different world, functioning night and day as Head of a suspect organisation, with the specific dual tasks of catching out my own predecessor and other senior subordinates as well as the professional smugglers, samsu distillers and other wrongdoers who had many of my staff in their pockets. I met with considerable success, partly due to the high rates of reward which we paid to informers . . . Some of the old hands did not even wait to be sacked. One produced a

276

medical certificate testifying that he was likely to die of sprue if he did not leave the tropics immediately, and sailed the same day! Another, who had failed to report to me, sent in a cavalier letter of resignation apologising for his shortcomings, saying he did not feel up to serving under a new Head. I do not think either of them troubled to draw their salaries, which had obviously been a very small portion of their income. . . .

But against the long term success in clearing up the department . . . there were many individual cases where we were outwitted by the astuteness of the smugglers. . . .

Information came in from a ship's officer that a number of sacks had been thrown overboard during the night from the stern of a ship some distance off the Horsburgh Lighthouse. Our launches went out but failed to find any trace. We later learned that the sacks were attached to small floats which only came to the surface a calculated number of hours later, when they were retrieved by a fast Japanese fishing boat which took their contents – tins of chandu worth $60,000 – to a hiding place at Tanah Merah Besar. Plans were now being made to bring the chandu into Singapore, where our recent successes had raised the black market price from under $4 to over $5 a tahil [about 1½ ounces].

Here was a test for the new broom. I was determined to block every approach to Singapore town and evolved what I thought was a complete blockade of Tanah Merah by land and sea. After three exhausting days and nights during which we earned considerable unpopularity . . . I realised that the blockade had failed, because the price of chandu dropped again to $3.80.

This is what happened, as we found out later. . . . The smugglers started off for Singapore with two large open cars. The leading car had very bright headlights and was full of well-dressed young Chinese. The chandu was in the second car, which showed no lights. As soon as he saw the Revenue Officers in the lights of the first car the driver of the second car, an ex-Revenue supervisor turned crook, pulled up . . . where there was a slight dip. The young Chinese in the first car were most co-operative and professed to be much amused at the idea of being searched for opium, suggesting taking the tyres off and opening up the engine. At last the search was over and with sarcastic farewells they drove off, halting, however, when they were out of sight . . . and hurrying back through the rubber and scrub whence they manhandled the chandu from the second to the first car. In due course the second car, now innocently empty, was also most thoroughly searched. Quite simple really – perhaps they deserved to get away with it!

ANDREW GILMOUR
An Eastern Cadet's Anecdotage (1974)

Glossary

Samshoo or **Samsu** – thrice fired. A general name among foreigners for Chinese fermented liquors of all kinds.

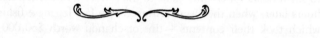

c.1939

The Night is Young

Australian newspaper-man, Ronald McKie, took a stroll through Chinatown one typical Saturday evening and absorbed the distinctive atmosphere of its street life.

Flickers of lightning miles away behind the white dome of the Malay mosque.

I am in a street that starts at a humped bridge near quays lined with godowns and ends half a mile away at the feet of a hospital. Along one side shop-houses, peeling and pock-marked in daylight, rise two and three storeys above celestial blue doorways to purple and scarlet balconies in the night light of deception; and in front, rows of food-stalls elbow each other into the roadway among the crowd which surges from alley-ways and doors and is pushed aside by nosing cars and jangling bicycle bells and the hoarse hoots of ricksha coolies.

There are probably twenty thousand people in this street who ignore the blaring truculent arguments of a hundred shop radios splitting the air in half a dozen languages, and above the din the shrill voice of a Chinese girl on a gramophone record is like an endless string of metal filings falling on an iron roof. She takes a high note and I wait for it to crash, while shuffling feet stir up the fine dust and send it drifting like smoke past fly-speckled electric light bulbs, and a waddling Chinese mother holds her child by the arms while it micturates into the gutter beside a food-stall.

The dust settles like grey talcum powder on the pink obscenity of plucked fowls hanging by the heels, on heaps of bloody guts and chunks of meat, on red crabs and silver fish, dried sea slugs strung up in hideous rows, cauldrons of steaming rice, platters of dates and dried figs, fruits in thick syrup, chopped bamboo shoots, smooth whiteness of perspiring onions, cooked white mice, slabs of shivering liver, dismembered chickens, something which might be the behind of a

279

puppy bulging with seasoning, garlic and sharks' fins and the crackling brown skin of ducks, heaps of days-old vegetables – all sweating and slobbering and slithering and dripping and exuding a combined smell like the local sanitary cart passing through the streets of a country town at high noon.

Cooks with hairless chests and glistening umbilicus-dented bellies and wide money belts of scarlet or brown or black holding up shorts or pantaloons stand before naked fires from coke stoves, hacking and slicing and stirring shallow red-hot iron dishes full of bubbling messes; they shout and spit through the steam, while assistants fill rows of cheap china bowls with moist rice and hand out unwashed chopsticks to hungry coolies who hold the bowls under their chins and shovel like animals and blow their noses among the heaps of vegetable cuttings.

It is a street of a dozen tongues, but the people are mostly Chinese and the noise is like the roar of a cup-final crowd gone crazy. A ricksha boy curses right and left as he drags his passenger through the surge, an old Chinese in black silk and skull cap and a few cultivated wisps of beard which are stroked lovingly; behind comes a permed and pomaded Chinese girl in an apricot-silk Shanghai gown, who lies back in her ricksha and languidly smokes a cigarette in a long holder and leaves a trail of heavy scent among the coolies and clerks and amahs and pick-pockets and gangster assistants.

Coolie women crocodile among the stinking stalls. Their faded blue coats and pants just below the knee, and wide straw hats over red bandana handkerchiefs tied under their chins, are smeared with clay and cement dust, and their stolid faces are the closest to earth of any women. They stop to eat their rice and belch in stall assistants' faces, and Chinese children with bare smeared bottoms weave among their legs and beg and steal and chew bone ends thrown at them by the laughing cooks.

Ice carriers chop slippery chunks on dirty boards, put the pieces into pink drinks made with brown water from dented buckets, sell water ices and toffee licks to the swarming kids who have sores in their hair and scabby necks, and I step like a wet cat through slime and banana skins and dollops of expectoration and excreta from squatting children, and walk along the road edge where shopkeepers scream their wares laid out in neat rows on the cement under the open sky.

I can buy belts, buckles, underpants, pencils, electric torches, lanterns, silks, nightgowns, boot polish, paint, sandals, pills, medicines, bottles of herbs, tins of ineffective contraceptives, safety-pins, bolts, gramophone records, scrap metal, paper flowers, shaving brushes, fountain pens, fly swatters, sarongs. Hundreds of yards of junk, thick with dust, product of civilizing factories; but nowhere could I find a roll of sanitary paper.

Sales men and women shout, cringe, flatter – any subterfuge to sell a fake sarong made in Osaka for three times its value, a pair of green clogs worth twenty cents for two dollars. The night is young and prices are high, but wait until the crowds start thinning and prices will fall like chips from a fruit machine when you ring the three aces. But I cannot wait. I buy a fly swatter for a few cents to whack blatant bottoms of kids whining for coppers – "No father no mother no makan no whisky soda" is one of the cries of the East's beggar children – and move down the road, away from the claptrap made by sweated workers in dingy, ill-lit, heavy-aired factories thousands of miles away where conditions should be better but are not. . . .

R.C.H. McKIE
This Was Singapore (1942)

1941

"Pigi Raffles"

After taking his university degree in Sydney, Russell Braddon volunteered to join the Australian Imperial Forces and was soon posted with his unit to Singapore. It was a move which would lead within months to active service and imprisonment by the Japanese; but he found that the arrival of the Australians was not universally welcomed.

After three weeks in Malaya we had none of us, we ordinary soldiers, spoken to a white woman (except the volunteers at the Anzac Club, who only had time to ask, "One lump or two?" as they poured one's tea). To address a European woman or girl – or in many cases, man – anywhere in Singapore (whether it was a shop, a cinema or in the street) was to incur the most calculated snub.

This was something we found impossible to combat and impossible to understand. Whilst one expected no gratitude for having been posted to Malaya, presumably to defend these quaint people, and whilst one expected no automatic hospitality (although one was very homesick and greatly longed for it), one nevertheless *did* expect civility. And civility was precisely what one did not, at any time, from any quarter, get. . . .

For my part, I received, from friends of my mother's, four invitations to go at any time to various estates on the mainland. From my grandmother I received two letters of introduction – one to the Governor of Singapore (this I considered hardly suitable, so I gave it to a rickshaw boy in the fond hope that he would use it) and another to the daughter of one of her greatest friends. This woman, my grandmother told me, always dined on Sundays at Raffles. "Go to Raffles and send this note in to her", the letter said, "but don't go by taxi because the native taxi drivers are Muslims and not afraid to die."

How well my grandmama knew Malayan taxi drivers. So I took a

282

rickshaw on my last Sunday leave in Singapore – we were due to go up-country the next week – and said firmly, "Raffles". And when I observed the boy, even more firmly, to be trotting off in the direction of Lavender Street, I leaped out of his rickshaw and, standing in front of him, bellowed: "Pigi, Raffles", *"Go to Raffles".* And as I climbed back into the seat, I added a thunderous: "Lacas!!" – *"quickly".* Astounded at my fluent command of the language, and not realizing that I had thus expended two-thirds of my total Malayan vocabulary, the boy meekly obeyed. Quite soon we were there. Having struck a hard bargain and paid the rickshaw off, I climbed the steps, ignored the "Out of Bounds" sign and entered the luxurious coolness of Singapore's most expensive hotel.

"Sir", the doorkeeper protested, and pointed at the "Out of Bounds" sign.

"Nuts", I told him – it was a word to which he was apparently not accustomed, for he relapsed into an uneasy silence whilst I straightened my slacks and saw that my hair was no untidier than usual. This done, I handed him my grandmother's letter. "Do you know this lady?" I asked, pointing at the address. "Yes, sir".

"Would you take the letter to her, please, and ask her if she can spare a minute – I'd like to see her if I may". "Yes, sir", said the doorkeeper – and vanished. After a few minutes, I tired of hanging around. I was thirsty and decided to get a drink. I walked into the lounge, sat down and ordered a long squash. And as I did so, a tall, fair-haired woman, thirty-ish and remarkably good-looking, strolled coolly into the room and sat down nearby.

"Boy", she called. The drinks-waiter came running. "Tell that soldier", she said in the clear, ringing tones of the very rich when talking about the very poor, whom they fondly imagine to be deaf, "that he's out of bounds in here and ask him to leave".

Obediently the "boy" pattered over. "You're out of bounds, sir", he said diffidently.

"Well, that's O.K. by me", I told him.

"But the lady . . ." protested the boy.

"Tell the lady", I answered rudely, "to go to hell".

The boy pattered back and relayed a mealy-mouthed version of my original. Promptly she reacted. Turning round to look at me for the first time – which she did with unconcealed distaste – she instructed the boy: "Go outside and call the Military Police", and then, as the boy was about to leave, added: "and while you're out there, bring in the Mr. Braddon who brought this note – ask him if he'll have a drink with me in here".

The opportunity was too good to miss. I walked over to her: "I'm Braddon", I said, "and I wouldn't drink here or anywhere else with you. And when this war with Japan starts and you go screeching off on the first evacuation ship to Australia, I sincerely hope that none of my family will either".

With that, feeling like Garrick on one of his best exits, I left. At the door she caught me.

"Mr Braddon", she began . . .

"Gunner Braddon", I interrupted.

"I'm awfully sorry", she continued, "must you go? Where are you going?"

"Lavender Street", I told her, "the Green Cat. Down there the women are bitches and they know it. I think I prefer it that way".

At that moment a provost arrived and so I – rather precipitately – left. Left her to explain why she'd summoned him. I just sat in my rickshaw as it headed down past the Great World towards the street of brothels and wondered why wars had to be so unpleasant. It was almost four years later that I heard that the fair-haired lady to whom I had carried my letter of introduction in Raffles was drowned when one of the *last* evacuee ships left Singapore Harbour. Apparently she had been very brave.

RUSSELL BRADDON
The Naked Island (1952)

My attack on Singapore was a bluff – a bluff that worked.
I had 30,000 men and was outnumbered more than three
to one. I knew that if I had to fight long for Singapore,
I would be beaten. That is why the surrender had to be
at once. I was very frightened all the time that the British
would discover our numerical weakness and lack of supplies
and force me into disastrous street fighting. (1942)

LIEUTENANT-GENERAL YAMASHITA TOMOYUKI
Commanding the 25th Japanese Army
(quoted in *A Soldier Must Hang* by John Deane Potter, 1963)

Glossary

Adelphi Hotel - first established in Raffles Place in 1863; later moved to High Street and finally to Coleman Street.

Amah - a nurse; from the Portuguese *ama*.

Amok *or* Amuck - a term used by Malays to signify an ungovernable state of mind, in which a desire to murder is predominant.

Attap - the dried leaf of the nipah palm, doubled over a small stick of bamboo, and thus used in the Malay peninsula for roofing houses.

Ayam - a generic name for fowls; a cock, a hen.

Baju - the upper portion of the Malay dress.

Bazaar - from the Persian *bazar* a market.

Bendahara - (Sanskrit bandahara) the title of a very high official in a Malay state - usually the highest in power outside the royal family; theoretically, the Treasurer.

Betel-nut - the leaf of the *sirih* or betelpepper smeared with chunam, or lime, and tobacco, and the nut of the areca palm, chewed together by the Chinese and other eastern nations.

Blakan Mati - now called Sentosa island.

Bugis, The - a race of people from the southern part of the island of Celebes . . . They are distinct from the Malays in point of language and in intelligence, though very similar in appearance.

Cære - *see* Sireh.

Campong - a Malay word meaning *enclosure*. Generally used for a *village*.

Campong Java - on the east coast near Bedok.

Celestial Empire - a common name for China, taken probably from the phrase Heavenly Dynasty, which has been for many centuries in use amongst the Chinese themselves . . . [Hence 'Celestials'].

Chandoo - (Malay) opium prepared for smoking.

Chetties - the usurers or money-lending section of the Klings.

Chop - a mark, number or brand.

Chota Hazri - the 'small breakfast,' or the early tea and toast . . . Corrupted form of the Hindi *chhoti hazri*.

Chunam - a Sanskrit word meaning *lime*. A mixture of lime, oil, and sand, used in China for paving yards, paths, racquet-courts, etc.

287

Clyde Terrace Market - built in Beach Road in 1872; demolished 1984.

Commercial Square - officially renamed Raffles Place in 1858.

Compradore - negotiator of purchases. From the Portuguese *comprar* to buy. The name given to the Chinese agent through whose means foreign merchants in China effect their purchases and sales.

Coolie - the menial of the east.

Cue - the tail of hair worn by every Chinaman. Introduced into China by the present (Manchu) dynasty only about 250 years ago . . . It is said to have been originally adopted by the Manchus in imitation of a horse's tail, as a graceful tribute to the animal to which they owed so much.

Damar *or* **Dammar** - a kind of resin dug out of the forests by the Malays . . . It is used by the Malays for torches, and by the Chinese for caulking boats.

Dhoby - the Hindi word (*dhobi*) for a washerman.

Duwit - (Dutch: duit) a cent, a doit; money in general. . . . now it is a name given . . . (in Singapore) to ¼ cent.

Fantan - the celebrated method of gambling with cash, common in China. . . . A pile of the coin is covered with a bowl, and the players stake on what the remainder will be when the heap has been divided by 4 - namely 1, 2, 3, nothing.

Forbidden Hill - Government Hill; after 1861 called Fort Canning Hill.

Fort Palmer - guarded the eastern entrance to New Harbour (N.B. Palmer Road).

Gaol - Outram Road Prison; built 1847, demolished 1968.

Gap - the Gap was a popular viewpoint at Pasir Panjang.

German Teutonia Club - its premises are now the Goodwood Park Hotel.

Gharry - a kind of four-wheeled carriage in use at Singapore. From the Hindi *gari*.

Godown - (1) originally a cellar or place to which it was necessary to *go down*. Now, a warehouse. (2) from the Malay *gedong*, a warehouse.

Government Hill - *see* Forbidden Hill.

Government House - on Government Hill up to 1869; the new Government House completed in 1869 is now the Istana Negara off Orchard Road.

Greater Town - China Town and business area south of Singapore River.

Hotel de l'Europe - on the corner of High Street facing the Padang; demolished in 1936 and replaced by the present Supreme Court building.

Jaga - Sanskrit. Wakefulness; the act of watching . . . orang jaga: a watchman.

Jinricksha *or* **Jinrikisha** - the man's strength cart. A small gig, invented about 1872 and constructed to carry one or more persons, drawn by a coolie in shafts and sometimes pushed by another from behind.

Johnston's Pier - erected c.1854 opposite the present Fullerton Building; demolished 1933. Named after Mr. A.L. Johnston who began trading in Singapore in 1819.

Joss – a Chinese idol; also applied to the Christian God. The word is a corruption of the Portuguese *Deos*, God, and has come to be used in pidgin-English in the sense of luck.

Junk – only the larger kind of Chinese sailing-vessels should be so called; but the term is now used of all sea-going boats and of the more bulky of the river craft. . . . Probably from the Malay *ajong* or *jong*, which means a large boat, corrupted by the Portuguese into *junco*.

Kambing – a generic name for sheep and goats.

Kampong – *see* Campong.

Kay-tow (Khehtow) – Head of the strangers. An employer of Chinese labour in the Straits.

Kelong – the well-known fish-trap everywhere seen on the shores of the Peninsula.

Keramat or Karamat – Arab. A saint, a holy place; a miracle working place, shrine or person, especially when the miracles are due to the personal sanctity of a living or dead man.

Klings, The – the common term in the Straits Settlements for all Indians.

Kolek – a Malay canoe; the small narrow boat with very sharp lines commonly known among Europeans as a 'koleh'.

K'ot'ou or Kow-tow or Kotoo – knock the head. The ceremony of prostration common in China.

Kris or Karis – pronounced *krees* or *creese*. A dagger of irregular shape, worn by the Malays in a sheath at the girdle. That a mere scratch may be effective, it is occasionally kept poisoned; and streaks of blood upon it are carefully preserved as honourable marks.

Lesser Town – native quarter north of Singapore River.

Li – about one third of a mile English.

London Hotel – started in Coleman Street in the 1840s; in 1845 moved to the site of the later Hotel de l'Europe.

Mace – the tenth part of a Chinese tael or ounce.

Makan – eating.

Makanan – food.

Mandarin – any Chinese official, civil or military, who wears a button (the knobs adopted by the Manchu dynasty to indicate rank . . .) may be so called. From the Portuguese *mandar* to command.

Meyer Mansion – on the corner of Coleman Street and North Bridge Road.

New Harbour – renamed Keppel Harbour in 1900.

Nyonyah – an appellation or title given . . . (in the Straits) to Straits-born Chinese and Eurasian ladies.

Pagar – a fence; a palisade; a row of stakes or palings.

Pahit – bitterness. [Hence a drink such as gin and bitters.]

Pakka (Pukkah) – a Hindi word meaning (1) ripe, cooked, and (2) genuine, proper. The application of this word in Anglo-Indian and Anglo-Chinese

289

parlance is practically unlimited. It is generally understood in the sense of 'real'.

Palanquin – a term applied in the Straits Settlements to four-wheeled close carriages.

Parang – a large Malay knife for cutting wood.

Passier Rice – Pasir Ris; a village on the northeast coast, opposite Pulau Ubin.

Penghulu – a chief, a headman.

Peon – one who serves on foot. A Singapore native constable.

Pigtail – *see* Cue.

Prahu *or* **Prau** – a Malay sea-going vessel, as opposed to a sampan.

Pukat – a seine-net, or drift net.

Pulo – the Malay word for *island*.

Punkah – a Hindi word (pankha) meaning a 'fan'.

Queue – *see* Cue.

Raja – a Sanskrit word meaning *king*.

Rickshaw – *see* Jinricksha.

Salah – fault, error, falling short.

Sambal – spices and other condiments eaten with curry to heighten the flavour.

Sampan – a Chinese boat of any kind, short of a junk, may be so called. From the Malay *sampan*, a small boat.

Sarong – part of the national costume of the Malays, consisting of an oblong cloth from 2 to 4 feet in width and about 2 yards in length. . . . It is invariably of a check pattern, generally in gay colours.

Sea View Hotel – a beach hotel at Tanjong Katong popular from the 1900s; demolished 1969.

Selat – a strait; an arm of the sea separating two pieces of land. . . . By extension, *selat* is a name often given to the Settlement of Singapore.

Singapore Club – an exclusive club established in 1861 in Cecil Street. Moved to Exchange Building overlooking the harbour in 1880; and again to Fullerton Building in 1927.

Sinkeh – new arrivals. Immigrant Chinese are so called in the Straits. They are much looked down upon by the Babas, or Straits-born Chinese, who are very proud of their nationality as British subjects.

Siranjong – the district of Serangoon.

Sireh – the betel-vine.

Stink-Pots – earthern jars, charged with materials of an offensive and suffocating smell, formerly much used by pirates . . . and a recognised weapon in Chinese warfare.

Syce (Sais) – a groom.

Tail – *see* Cue.

Tanjong – a cape; a head-land, a promontory.

Temenggong – the title of an exalted Malay official.

Tiffin – the mid-day meal; luncheon. From the Persian *tafannun*.

Tongkang – a kind of lighter or cargo-boat.

Towkay – Head of the house. The common term in the Swatow and Amoy districts for *master*, whether of a family or shop.

Town Hall – now the Victoria Theatre in Empress Place.

Tuan Besar – 'Great master', or head of the establishment. Used in the Straits much as *Sahib* in India. (Malay).

Union Hotel – in North Bridge Road.

van Wijk Hotel – in Stamford Road.

Wang – money; a small coin, = (about) 2½ cents.

Whampoa Gardens – pleasure gardens on the road to Serangoon; developed and owned by Hoo Ah Kay (1816–1880) who came from Whampoa near Canton in China.

HERBERT A. GILES
A Glossary of Reference on Subjects connected with the Far East (1878)

R.J. WILKINSON
A Malay-English Dictionary (1901)

and a glossary of place names by Michael Wise.

Events

1819	Sir Stamford Raffles lands
	First treaty signed with Malay rulers
	William Farquhar appointed Resident
1821	Census shows population now 4,727
1822	First Government House erected on Forbidden Hill
	First bridge opened across Singapore River
1823	John Crawfurd appointed Resident
	Raffles leaves Singapore for last time
	Census shows population now 10,683
1824	*Singapore Chronicle* begins publication
	Final treaty signed with Malay rulers
	Singapore becomes British settlement
1827	First steamship is seen at Singapore
1833	Census shows population now 20,978
1834	First New Year Regatta
1836	Completion of Armenian Church
1837	Chamber of Commerce formed
1839	Launching of first Singapore-built vessel
1840	Opening of first bank: Union Bank of Calcutta
	Census shows population now 33,969
1843	First race meeting held
1845	Opening of first Masonic Lodge
	Straits Times begins publication
	Arrival of first P & O mail boat
1850	Census shows population now 52,891
	Visit of the Governor-General of India, the Marquess of Dalhousie
1851	Horsburgh Lighthouse commences operation
1854	Serious Chinese riots
1859	Construction of Fort Canning begins
1860	Telegraph opened between Singapore and Batavia
	Census shows population now 81,734
1862	St. Andrew's Cathedral opened and consecrated

1864	First use of gas street lighting
1865	Coleman Bridge opened
1867	Transfer of Straits Settlements from Indian administration to become Crown Colony
1869	Opening of Suez Canal Building of Government House completed
1871	Inaugural meeting of Singapore Railway Company Visit of the King of Siam Telegraph opened between Singapore and Hong Kong Census shows population now 94,816
1877	Rubber first introduced into Malaya Formation of Straits Branch, Royal Asiatic Society Hongkong & Shanghai Bank opens Singapore branch
1879	General Ulysses Grant visits Singapore Building of Masonic Hall, Coleman Street, commenced Opening of Singapore Club, Chamber of Commerce and Exchange Building First official postcards issued by Straits Settlements Postal Department
1880	Jinrikishas introduced from Shanghai
1881	Opening of Telephone Exchange Census shows population now 137,722 Formation of Yacht Club
1882	Visit of Prince Albert Victor and Prince George of Wales
1883	Telephone service extended to Johore
1886	Last horse sales in Raffles Place Steam trams begin operation Ord Bridge opened
1887	Golden Jubilee Celebrations for Queen Victoria Unveiling of Raffles Statue Photographic Society formed
1889	Cycling Club established
1891	Singapore Golf Club formed First concert by Philharmonic Society Census shows population now 181,602
1892	Pulau Bukum petrol tank station opened
1894	Picture postcards begin to be used on a large scale
1896	Sultan Shoal Lighthouse commences operation
1897	Diamond Jubilee Celebrations for Queen Victoria Installation of electric light at Tanjong Pagar Wharves
1900	New Harbour renamed Keppel Harbour
1901	Death of Queen Victoria Visit of Duke and Duchess of Cornwall

1901	Census shows population now 226,842
1903	Singapore-Kranji railway opened
1904	Registration of motorcars and testing and licensing of drivers introduced
1905	First supply of cold storage goods received Electric trams commence operation Victoria Memorial Hall opened
1906	One dollar currency notes introduced
1907	Formation of Singapore Automobile Club
1909	Victoria Theatre completed
1911	Census shows population now 303,321
1914	Outbreak of the Great War in Europe
1915	Singapore Mutiny
1921	Slump in rubber industry Census shows population now 418,358
1922	Visit of Prince of Wales Malaya Borneo Exhibition held
1923	Opening of Johore Causeway
1926	First trolley bus service introduced
1928	Start of Singapore Flying Club Chinese in Singapore begin Japanese boycott
1929	Direct telegraphic link London-Singapore established
1930	Amy Johnson arrives on solo England-Australia flight Worst year in the history of the rubber industry
1931	London-Singapore airmail takes 10 days Census shows population now 570,128
1935	Silver Jubilee of George V: Sultan of Johore donates £½m for Singapore defences
1936	Anti-Japanese riots by Chinese begin in Singapore Start of wireless broadcasting
1937	Sultan Mosque installs loudspeakers for muezzin's call to prayer Kallang aerodrome opened Proceeds from opium sales still providing 25% of Straits Settlements' budget
1938	Inauguration of Singapore Naval Base (cost £9m) First set of synchronised traffic lights installed
1939	World War II begins in Europe
1941	Japan invades Malaya Sinking of *Prince of Wales* and *Repulse*
1942	Japan takes Singapore
1945	Japanese surrender

Acknowledgements

Grateful acknowledgements are due to the following publishers, authors and others:

W.H. Allen & Co. Ltd.
Reminiscences of an Indian Official by General Sir Orfeur Cavenagh

A & C Black Ltd.
Wanderings in South-Eastern Seas by Charlotte Cameron

Chapman & Hall Ltd.
The Rambles of a Globe-Trotter by E.K. Laird

J.M. Dent & Sons Ltd.
An Eastern Voyage by Count Fritz von Hochberg

Dodd, Mead & Company, Inc.
A Beachcomber in the Orient by Harry L. Foster

Harper & Row, Publishers, Inc.
My Last Cruise by A.W. Habersham
Around the World: Sketches of Travel by E.D.G. Prime

Harrap Ltd.
Singapore Patrol by Alec Dixon

Hutchinson Publishing Group Limited
Malayan Symphony by W. Robert Foran
In British Malaya Today by Richard J.H. Sidney
Footprints in Malaya by Sir Frank Swettenham

Longman Group Ltd.
A Voyage in the "Sunbeam" by Mrs. Brassey
A Lady's Second Journey Round the World by Ida Pfeiffer

Macmillan Publishers Ltd.
The Cruise of Her Majesty's Ship "Bacchante" 1879-1882 by Prince Albert Victor and Prince George of Wales
The Malay Archipelago by Alfred Russel Wallace

Malaya Publishing House
Musings of JSMR mostly Malayan by J.S.M. Rennie
Singapura Sorrows by R.N. Walling

Methuen & Co. Ltd. together with **Mr. Thomas L. Braddell** and **O.U.P.**
The Lights of Singapore by Roland Braddell

John Murray (Publishers) Ltd.
About Others and Myself by Major-General Sir Archibald Anson
The Golden Chersonese by Isabella L. Bird
Scented Isles and Coral Gardens by C.D. MacKellar
Sunny Lands and Seas by Hugh Wilkinson
One Hundred Years of Singapore edited by Walter Makepeace, Gilbert Brooke and
Roland Braddell

Putnam together with **Mr. Robin Bruce Lockhart** and **Campbell Thomson &
McLaughlin Ltd.**
Return to Malaya by R.H. Bruce Lockhart

Routledge & Kegan Paul PLC
Two Years in the Jungle by William T. Hornaday

Sampson Low
Our New Way Round the World by Charles Carleton Coffin
Looking for Luck by James Redfern
The Straits of Malacca, Indo-China and China by J. Thomson
The Land of the White Elephant by Frank Vincent, Jun.

Charles Scribner's Sons
Round the World by Andrew Carnegie
Where the Strange Trails Go Down by E. Alexander Powell

Thacker & Co. Ltd.
Why Singapore Fell by Lieut.-Gen. H. Gordon Bennett

The Malaysian Branch of The Royal Asiatic Society
Letters of Colonel Nahuijs translated by H.E. Miller

The Straits Times
Extracts from 1883 and 1942

The Times of London
Extracts from 1915, 1921 and 1923

Whitcoulls Ltd.
Letters written to my Children by Edward G. Lane

Singapore: the Japanese Version by Colonel Masanobu Tsuji, translated by Margaret E.
Lake (unfortunately it has not proved possible to trace the copyright holder of this
work)

The National Library, Singapore and the **National University of Singapore
Library** for access to their South East Asian collections

Rhodes House Library, Oxford for permission to quote from Otto Ziegele's
manuscript diary

The Swiss Club, Singapore for permission to quote from H.R. Arbenz's
manuscript memoir

Chang Chin Chiang for permission to quote from his translation of Li Chung
Chu's *Description of Singapore in 1887*

Lim Kheng Chye, Andrew Tan Kim Guan, Paul Yap Kong Meng, and the
Archives & Oral History Department, Singapore for the use of Picture
Postcards from their collections

Andrew Gilmour C.M.G., **G.L. Peet, Fawzia Talbert,** and **Ray Tyers** for advice and assistance

Mun Him Wise for research, guidance and much hard work.

Tale-end

A.P. Watt
Extract from *From Sea to Sea and Other Sketches* by Rudyard Kipling reproduced by permission of A.P. Watt Ltd. on behalf of the National Trust for Places of Historic Interest or Natural Beauty.

The Trustees of the late Lady Sarah Winstedt's Will Trust
For permission to quote from Sir Richard Winstedt's *Start from Alif: Count from One*.

Dr Alan Gilmour, CVO, CBE and Mr Andrew Gilmour
For permission to quote from their late father's *An Eastern Cadet's Anecdotage*.

Robert Hale Ltd
This was Singapore by R.C.H. McKie.

Curtis Brown
Extract from *The Naked Island* reproduced with permission of Curtis Brown Ltd, London on behalf of Russell Braddon. Copyright © 1952.

If any other acknowledgements are due but have been overlooked, the Compiler offers his sincere apologies.

297

Index

298

299

Michael Wise was born in London in 1937 and is a graduate of Oxford University where he obtained an MA in Philosophy, Politics and Economics. His subsequent business career took him overseas, particularly to the East, and he was resident in Singapore for a number of years.

His historical and literary interests led him to pursue the travel literature of the countries where he worked, and in 1985 his first collection – *Travellers' Tales of Old Singapore* – was published by Times Books International. Since then, three more of his collections of oriental travel writing have been published. Michael Wise now lives in England with his Singapore-born wife.

Michael Wise
Travellers' Tales of Old Hong Kong
(ISBN 1 873047 86 X)

Here are the exploits and escapades of travellers from around
the world, set in Hong Kong and the neighbouring South
China coast. Drawn from personal memoirs, letters and
diaries, this collection spans more than a century – from
the years before Britain took formal possession of Hong Kong
to the time of the Japanese occupation.

A recurrent theme in their often racy and humorous stories is
the never ending battle of wits between Chinese and foreigners
as they seek to address a host of East/West misunderstandings.
Vividly told, the *Tales* are by turns informative or astounding,
moving or amusing, but always entertaining.

*   *   *

True Tales of British India
(ISBN 1 873047 06 1)

A collection of tales brimming with humour, surprises, and
insight. Guided by a succession of stimulating companions
the reader is conveyed from the drawing rooms of Simla to the
slums of Calcutta; from the North West Frontier to Cox's
Bazaar, with many a detour and excitement along the way.

**". . . a great deal of humour and adventure. . . . This is not a
book to make one feel proud of the British Raj, but it is still
fascinating. Consisting of some 70 or more well-chosen
reminiscences, it is an excellent book for reading on a
crowded train journey or on a hot summer's day when ice
tinkles in the G&T. The glossary of Indian terms, the
chronological table, and a competent index, add to the
book's value."** *Concord* – Journal of the English Speaking
Union of the Commonwealth

"A terrific collection . . ." *The Good Book Guide*

These books are compiled by Michael Wise and published by
In Print Publishing Ltd, 9 Beaufort Terrace, Brighton BN2 2SU.
Tel: +44 1273 682 836. Fax: +44 1273 620958